*Quick*FACTS™

Breast CANCER

What You Need to Know—NOW

*Quick*FACTS™

From the Experts at the American Cancer Society

Breast
CANCER

What You Need to Know—NOW

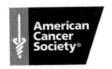

Published by the American Cancer Society/Health Promotions
250 Williams Street NW, Atlanta, Georgia 30303 USA

Printed in the United States of America
Cover designed by Jill Dible, Atlanta, GA
Edited by Jennifer L. Sharpe, Wilson, NC
Composition by Graphic Composition, Inc., Bogart, GA

5 4 3 2 1   11 12 13 14 15

Library of Congress Cataloging-in-Publication Data

Quick facts breast cancer: what you need to know—now /
from the experts at the American Cancer Society.
  p. cm. — (Quickfacts)
  title: Breast cancer : what you need to know—now
  Includes bibliographical references and index.
  ISBN-13: 978-1-60443-031-8 (pbk. : alk. paper)
  ISBN-10: 1-60443-031-1 (pbk. : alk. paper)
  1. Breast—Cancer—Popular works. I. American Cancer
Society. II. Title: Breast cancer : what you need to know—now.
RC280.B8Q52 2011
616.99'449—dc22

                                        2010028248

A Note to the Reader

This information represents the views of the doctors and
nurses serving on the American Cancer Society's Cancer
Information Database Editorial Board. These views are based
on their interpretation of studies published in medical journals,
as well as their own professional experience.

The treatment information in this book is not official policy of
the Society and is not intended as medical advice to replace the
expertise and judgment of your cancer care team. It is intended
to help you and your family make informed decisions, together
with your doctor.

Your doctor may have reasons for suggesting a treatment plan
different from these general treatment options. Don't hesitate to
ask him or her questions about your treatment options.

For more information, contact your American Cancer Society
at **800-227-2345** or **cancer.org**.

Quantity discounts on bulk purchases of this book are avail-
able. Book excerpts can also be created to fit specific needs.
For information, please contact the American Cancer Society,
Health Promotions Publishing, 250 Williams Street NW,
Atlanta, GA 30303-1002, or send an e-mail to **trade.sales@
cancer.org**.

TABLE OF CONTENTS

Diagnosis and Staging

Treatment

Your Breast Cancer

What Is Cancer?

The body is made up of hundreds of millions of living cells. Normal body cells grow, divide, and die in an orderly fashion. During the early years of a person's life, normal cells divide faster to allow the person to grow. After the person becomes an adult, most cells divide only to replace worn-out or dying cells or to repair injuries.

Cancer* begins when **cells** in a part of the body start to grow out of control. There are many kinds of cancer, but they all start because of out-of-control growth of abnormal cells.

Cancer cell growth is different from normal cell growth. Instead of dying, cancer cells continue to grow and form new, abnormal cells. Cancer cells can also invade (grow into) other tissues, something that normal cells cannot do. Growing out of control and invading other tissues are what makes a cell a cancer cell.

Cells become cancer cells because of damage to **DNA**. DNA is in every cell and directs all its

*Terms in bold are further explained in the Glossary, beginning on page 261.

actions. In a normal cell, when DNA becomes damaged, the cell either repairs the damage or the cell dies. In cancer cells, the damaged DNA is not repaired, but the cell doesn't die like it should. Instead, this cell goes on making new cells that the body does not need. These new cells will all have the same damaged DNA as the first cell.

People can inherit damaged DNA, but most DNA damage is caused by mistakes that happen while the normal cell is reproducing or by something in the environment. Sometimes the cause of the DNA damage is obvious, such as cigarette smoking. But often no clear cause is found.

In most cases, the cancer cells form a **tumor**. Some cancers, like **leukemia**, rarely form tumors. Instead, these cancer cells involve the blood and blood-forming organs and circulate through other tissues where they grow.

Cancer cells often travel to other parts of the body, where they begin to grow and form new tumors that replace normal **tissue**. This process is called **metastasis**. It happens when the cancer cells get into the bloodstream or lymph vessels of the body.

No matter where a cancer may spread, it is always named for the place where it started. For example, breast cancer that has spread to the liver is still called breast cancer, not liver cancer. Likewise, prostate cancer that has spread to the bone is metastatic prostate cancer, not bone cancer.

Different types of cancer can behave very differently. For example, lung cancer and breast cancer are very different diseases. They grow at different rates and respond to different treatments. That is why people with cancer need treatment that is aimed at their particular kind of cancer.

Not all tumors are cancerous. Tumors that aren't cancer are called **benign**. **Benign tumors** can cause problems—they can grow very large and press on healthy organs and tissues. But they cannot grow into (invade) other tissues. Because they can't invade, they also can't spread to other parts of the body (**metastasize**). These tumors are almost never life threatening.

What Is Breast Cancer?

Breast cancer is a malignant tumor that starts from cells of the **breast**. A **malignant tumor** is a group of cancer cells that may grow into (invade) surrounding tissues or spread (metastasize) to distant areas of the body. The disease occurs almost entirely in women, but men can get it, too.

The remainder of this book refers only to breast cancer in women. For information on breast cancer in men, contact your American Cancer Society at 800-227-2345 to request the document *Breast Cancer in Men*, or visit our Web site, **cancer.org**.

The Normal Breast

To understand breast cancer, it helps to have some basic knowledge about the normal structure of the breasts.

The female breast is made up mainly of **lobules** (milk-producing glands), **ducts** (tiny tubes that carry the milk from the lobules to the **nipple**), and **stroma** (fatty tissue and connective tissue surrounding the ducts and lobules, **blood vessels**, and lymphatic vessels).

Most breast cancers begin in the cells that line the ducts (**ductal carcinoma**). Some begin in the cells that line the lobules (**lobular carcinoma**), whereas a small number start in other tissues.

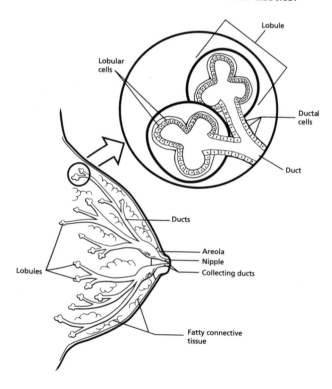

The lymph (lymphatic) system

The **lymphatic system** is important to understand because it is one of the ways in which breast cancers can spread. This system has several parts.

Lymph nodes are small, bean-shaped collections of immune system cells (cells that are important in fighting infections) that are connected by lymphatic vessels. **Lymphatic vessels** are like small veins. But instead of carrying blood as veins do, lymphatic vessels carry **lymph**, a clear fluid. Lymph contains tissue fluid and waste products, as well as immune system cells. Breast cancer cells can enter lymphatic vessels and begin to grow in lymph nodes.

Most lymphatic vessels in the breast connect to lymph nodes under the arm (**axillary lymph nodes**). Some lymphatic vessels connect to lymph nodes inside the chest (**internal mammary lymph nodes**) and to those either above or below the collarbone (**supraclavicular** or **infraclavicular lymph nodes**).

Knowing whether the cancer cells have spread to lymph nodes is important. If they have, there is a higher chance that the cells could have entered the bloodstream and metastasized (spread) to other sites in the body. The more lymph nodes that contain breast cancer, the more likely cancer will be found in other organs. The extent of the metastasis is important and will affect your treatment plan. Still, not all women with cancer cells in their lymph nodes will have metastasis, and, in some cases, a woman can have negative lymph nodes and still develop metastasis.

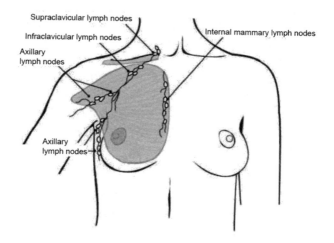

Benign Breast Lumps

Most breast lumps are benign (not cancerous). However, tissue samples may need to be taken from the lumps and viewed under a microscope to prove they are not cancerous.

Fibrocystic changes

Most lumps in the breast represent **fibrocystic changes**. Fibrocystic refers to fibrosis and cysts. Fibrosis is the formation of fibrous (scar-like) tissue, and **cysts** are fluid-filled sacs. Fibrocystic changes can cause breast swelling and pain. These changes often occur just before the start of your menstrual period. Your breasts may feel lumpy and you may notice a clear or slightly cloudy **nipple discharge**.

Other benign breast lumps

Benign breast tumors such as **fibroadenomas** or **intraductal papillomas** are abnormal growths, but they are not cancerous and do not spread outside of the breast to other organs. Benign breast tumors are not life threatening. Still, women who have certain benign breast conditions are at greater risk for developing breast cancer.

For more information about benign breast conditions see the section, "What Are the Risk Factors for Breast Cancer?" on pages 17–34. For more information on noncancerous breast conditions, contact your American Cancer Society at **800-227-2345** and request the document *Non-cancerous Breast Conditions*, or visit our Web site, **cancer.org**.

General Breast Cancer Terms

Following are some of the key words used to describe breast cancer.

Carcinoma

Carcinoma is a term for cancer that begins in the lining (**epithelial cells**) of organs such as the breast. Nearly all types of breast cancer are carcinomas (either ductal carcinomas or lobular carcinomas).

Adenocarcinoma

An **adenocarcinoma** is a type of carcinoma that starts in **glandular tissue** (tissue that makes and secretes a substance). The ducts and lobules of the breast are glandular tissue (they make breast milk), so cancers starting in these areas are often called adenocarcinomas.

Carcinoma in situ

Carcinoma in situ describes the early stage of cancer, when it is confined to the layer of cells where it began. In breast cancer, **in situ** means that the cancer cells remain confined to ducts (ductal carcinoma in situ) or lobules (lobular carcinoma in situ). The cells have not invaded deeper tissues in the breast or spread to other organs; therefore, this type of cancer is sometimes referred to as **noninvasive** or **preinvasive breast cancer**.

Invasive (infiltrating) carcinoma

An invasive (infiltrating) cancer is one that has grown beyond the layer of cells where it started (as opposed to carcinoma in situ). Most breast cancers are invasive carcinomas—either invasive ductal carcinoma or invasive lobular carcinoma.

Sarcoma

Sarcomas are cancers that start from connective tissues such as muscle tissue, fat tissue, or blood vessels. Sarcomas of the breast are rare.

Types of Breast Cancer

There are several types of breast cancer, some of which are quite rare. In some cases, a single breast tumor can have a combination of different types of cancerous cells or have a mixture of invasive and in situ cancer.

Ductal carcinoma in situ

Ductal carcinoma in situ (**DCIS**; also known as **intraductal carcinoma**) is the most common type of noninvasive breast cancer. DCIS means that the cancer cells are inside the ducts but have not spread through the walls of the ducts into the surrounding breast tissue.

About 1 in 5 new breast cancer cases will be DCIS. Nearly all women whose breast cancer is diagnosed at this early stage can be cured. A mammogram is often the best way to find DCIS early.

When DCIS is diagnosed, the pathologist will examine the tissue sample and look for **tumor necrosis** (dead or decaying cancer cells). If necrosis is present, the tumor is likely to be more aggressive. The term **comedocarcinoma** is often used to describe DCIS with necrosis.

Lobular carcinoma in situ

Lobular carcinoma in situ (**LCIS**; also called **lobular neoplasia**) is not a true cancer, but it is sometimes classified as a type of noninvasive breast cancer. It begins in the milk-producing glands but does not grow through the wall of the lobules.

Most breast cancer specialists believe that LCIS itself does not often become an invasive cancer. However, in women with this condition, there is a higher risk for invasive breast cancer to develop in the same breast or the other breast. For this reason, women with LCIS should have regular mammograms and doctor visits.

Invasive ductal carcinoma

Invasive (or infiltrating) **ductal carcinoma** (IDC) is the most common type of breast cancer, occurring in about 8 of 10 invasive breast cancers. IDC starts in a duct (or milk passage) of the breast, breaks through the wall of the duct, and grows into the fatty tissue of the breast. At this point, it may spread to other parts of the body through the lymphatic system and bloodstream.

Invasive lobular carcinoma

Invasive (or infiltrating) **lobular carcinoma (ILC)** starts in the lobules (milk-producing glands). Like IDC, it can metastasize to other parts of the body. About 1 in 10 invasive breast cancers is an invasive lobular carcinoma. Invasive lobular carcinoma may be harder to detect through mammography than invasive ductal carcinoma.

Less common types of breast cancer

Inflammatory breast cancer: This uncommon type of invasive breast cancer accounts for about 1% to 3% of all breast cancers. Usually, there is no single lump or tumor. Instead, **inflammatory breast cancer (IBC)** makes the skin of the breast look red and feel warm and gives the skin a thick, pitted appearance that resembles an orange peel. Doctors now know that these changes are not caused by inflammation or infection, but by cancer cells blocking lymphatic vessels in the skin. The affected breast may become larger, firmer, tender, or itchy. In its early stages, inflammatory breast cancer is often mistaken for an infection in the breast (called **mastitis**). Often, this cancer is first treated as an infection with antibiotics. If the symptoms are caused by cancer, they will not improve, and the skin may be biopsied to look for cancer cells. Because there is no actual lump, it may not be detected on a mammogram, which may make it even more difficult to find early. IBC tends to have a higher chance of spreading and a worse **prognosis** (outlook) than invasive ductal or lobular cancer.

For more information on inflammatory breast cancer, contact your American Cancer Society at **800-227-2345** and request the document *Inflammatory Breast Cancer*, or visit our Web site, **cancer.org**.

Triple-negative breast cancer: This term is used to describe breast cancers (usually invasive ductal carcinomas) in which the cells lack **estrogen receptors** and **progesterone receptors**. These cancer cells also do not have an excess of the **HER2 protein** on their surfaces. HER2 is a protein found on the surface of certain cancer cells. It is made by a specific gene called the HER2/neu gene.

Triple-negative breast cancers tend to occur more frequently in younger women and in black women and tend to grow and spread more quickly than other types of breast cancer. Because the tumor cells lack these estrogen and progesterone receptors, neither hormone therapy nor drugs that target HER2 are effective against these cancers (although chemotherapy can still be useful).

(See the section "How Is Breast Cancer Diagnosed?", page 86, for more detail on estrogen and progesterone receptors.)

Mixed tumors: Mixed tumors contain a variety of cell types, such as invasive ductal carcinoma combined with invasive lobular carcinoma. In this situation, the tumor is treated as if it were an invasive ductal carcinoma.

Medullary carcinoma: This special type of infiltrating breast cancer has a rather well-defined boundary between tumor tissue and normal tissue. It also has some other special features, including large cancer cells and the presence of immune system cells at the edges of the tumor. Medullary carcinoma accounts for about 3% to 5% of all breast cancers. The prognosis for this kind of breast cancer is generally better than that of the more common types of invasive breast cancer. Most cancer specialists believe true medullary carcinoma is very rare, and that the treatment approach for this cancer type should be the same as that for invasive ductal carcinoma.

Metaplastic carcinoma: Metaplastic carcinoma (also known as carcinoma with metaplasia) is a very rare type of invasive ductal carcinoma. These tumors include cells that normally are not found in the breast, such as cells that look like skin cells (squamous cells) or cells that make bone. These tumors are treated like invasive ductal carcinoma.

Mucinous carcinoma: Also known as colloid carcinoma, this rare type of invasive ductal carcinoma forms from abnormal cells that are in mucin, a component of mucus. Although many types of breast cancer produce mucus, in mucinous carcinoma the mucus forms part of the tumor. The prognosis for mucinous carcinoma is usually better than that for the more common types of invasive breast cancer. Still, it is treated like invasive ductal carcinoma.

Paget disease of the nipple: This type of breast cancer starts in the breast ducts and spreads to the skin of the nipple and then to the **areola**, the dark circle around the nipple. It is rare, accounting for only about 1% of all breast cancers. The skin of the nipple and areola often appears crusted, scaly, and red, with areas of bleeding or oozing. The woman may notice burning or itching.

Paget disease is almost always associated with either ductal carcinoma in situ (DCIS) or, more often, with invasive ductal carcinoma. Treatment often requires mastectomy. If only DCIS is found (with no invasive cancer) when the breast is removed, the prognosis is excellent.

Tubular carcinoma: Tubular carcinoma is another unique type of invasive ductal carcinoma. This type of carcinoma is called "tubular" because of the way the cells appear when seen under the microscope. Tubular carcinomas account for about 2% of all breast cancers and tend to have a better prognosis than most invasive ductal or lobular carcinomas.

Papillary carcinoma: The cells of papillary carcinomas tend to be arranged in small, finger-like projections when viewed under the microscope. These tumors can be separated into noninvasive and invasive types. Intraductal papillary carcinoma or papillary carcinoma in situ is noninvasive. It is often considered a subtype of ductal carcinoma in situ (DCIS) and is treated accordingly. In rare cases, papillary carcinoma is invasive, in which case it is treated like invasive ductal carcinoma, although the prognosis is likely to be better. Papillary carcinomas tend to be diagnosed in older women and make up no more than 2% of all breast cancers.

Adenoid cystic carcinoma (adenocystic carcinoma): Adenoid cystic carcinomas (ACCs) have both glandular (adenoid) and cylinder-like (cystic) features when seen under the microscope. They make up less than 1% of all breast cancers. ACCs rarely spread to the lymph nodes or distant areas and usually have a very good prognosis.

Phyllodes tumor: This very rare breast tumor is also called a phyllodes tumor or cytosarcoma phyllodes. It develops in the stroma (connective tissue) of the breast, in contrast to carcinomas, which develop in the ducts or lobules. Phyllodes tumors are usually benign but on rare occasions may be malignant.

Benign phyllodes tumors are treated by removing the mass along with a **margin** of normal breast tissue. Malignant phyllodes tumors are treated by removing the mass along with a wider margin of normal tissue or by **mastectomy**. Although surgery is often all that is needed, these cancers may not respond as well to the other treatments used for more common types of breast cancer. When a malignant phyllodes tumor has spread, it may be treated with the chemotherapy given for soft-tissue sarcomas. For more information on soft-tissue sarcomas, contact your American Cancer Society at **800-227-2345** and request the document *Sarcoma—Adult Soft Tissue Cancer*, or visit our Web site, **cancer.org**.

Angiosarcoma: Angiosarcoma starts from cells that line blood vessels or lymphatic vessels. It rarely occurs in the breast. When it does, it is usually seen as a complication of radiation treatment to the breast and often develops about 5 to 10 years after **radiation treatment**. However, this is an extremely rare complication of breast radiation therapy. Angiosarcoma can also occur in the arm of women who develop lymphedema as a result of lymph node surgery or radiation therapy used to treat breast cancer. (For information on lymphedema, see page 127 and pages 209–211.) Angiosarcomas tend to grow and spread quickly. Treatment is generally the same as that for other sarcomas.

For more information on sarcomas, contact your American Cancer Society at **800-227-2345** to request the document *Sarcoma—Adult Soft Tissue Cancer*, or visit our Web site, **cancer.org**.

What Are the Key Statistics About Breast Cancer?

Breast cancer is the most common cancer among American women, except for skin cancers. The chance of invasive breast cancer developing at some time in a woman's life is a little less than 1 in 8 (12%).

The American Cancer Society's most recent estimates for breast cancer in the United States are for 2010:

- About 207,090 new cases of invasive breast cancer will be diagnosed in women.

- About 54,010 new cases of carcinoma in situ (CIS) will be diagnosed (CIS is noninvasive and is the earliest stage of breast cancer).
- About 39,840 women will die of breast cancer.

After increasing for more than 2 decades, female breast cancer incidence rates decreased by about 2% per year from 1998 to 2007. This decrease was seen only in women aged 50 or older and may be due at least in part to the decline in use of hormone therapy after menopause that occurred after the results of the **Women's Health Initiative** were published in 2002. The Women's Health Initiative linked the use of hormone therapy to an increased risk of breast cancer and heart diseases.

Breast cancer is the second leading cause of cancer death in women, exceeded only by lung cancer. The chance that breast cancer will be responsible for a woman's death is about 1 in 35 (about 3%). Death rates from breast cancer have been declining since about 1990, with larger decreases in women younger than 50. These decreases are believed to be the result of earlier detection through screening and increased awareness, as well as improved treatment.

At this time, there are more than 2.5 million breast cancer survivors in the United States. (This figure includes women still being treated and those who have completed treatment.) Survival rates are discussed in the section "How Is Breast Cancer Staged?" on pages 106–107.

Risk Factors and Causes

What Are the Risk Factors for Breast Cancer?

A **risk factor** is anything that affects your chance of getting a disease, such as cancer. Different types of cancer have different risk factors. For example, exposing skin to strong sunlight is a risk factor for skin cancer. Smoking is a risk factor for cancers of the lung, mouth, larynx (voice box), bladder, kidney, and several other organs.

But risk factors don't tell us everything. Having a risk factor, or even several, does not mean that you will get the disease. Most women who have one or more breast cancer risk factors never get breast cancer, whereas many women with breast cancer have no apparent risk factors (other than being a woman and growing older). Even when breast cancer develops in a woman with risk factors, it is hard to know just how much these factors contributed.

There are different kinds of risk factors. Some factors, like a person's age or race, can't be changed. Others are linked to cancer-causing elements in the environment. Still others are related to personal behaviors, such as smoking, drinking, and diet. Some factors influence risk more than others, and a woman's risk for breast cancer can change over time because of aging or changes in lifestyle.

Risk Factors You Cannot Change

Gender

Simply being a woman is the main risk factor for breast cancer. Breast cancer can develop in men, but the disease is about 100 times more common among women. Although women have many more breast cells than men, the main reason breast cancer is more prevalent in women is because women's breast cells are constantly exposed to the growth-promoting effects of the female hormones **estrogen** and **progesterone**.

Aging

The risk of breast cancer increases as a woman gets older. About 1 in 8 invasive breast cancers is found in women younger than age 45, whereas about 2 of 3 invasive breast cancers are found in women aged 55 or older.

Genetic risk factors

About 5% to 10% of breast cancer cases are thought to be hereditary, resulting directly from **gene** defects (called **mutations**) inherited from a parent. For more information on genes and DNA, see the section, "Do We Know What Causes Breast Cancer?" on page 35.

BRCA1 and BRCA2: The most common causes of hereditary breast cancer are inherited mutations in the **BRCA1** or **BRCA2** genes. In normal cells, these genes help prevent cancer by making proteins that keep cells from growing abnormally. If you have **inherited** a mutated copy of either gene from a parent, you are at increased risk for breast cancer. Women with an inherited BRCA1 or BRCA2 mutation have up to an 80% chance of breast cancer developing during their lifetimes (often at a younger age than women not born with one of these gene mutations). These cancers are more often bilateral (occurring in both breasts) than cancers in women who do not have one of the gene mutations. Women with these inherited mutations also are at increased risk for other cancers, particularly ovarian cancer.

In the United States, BRCA mutations are found most often in Jewish women of Ashkenazi (Eastern European) origin, but they are also found in black and Hispanic women and can occur in any racial or ethnic group.

Changes in other genes: Other gene mutations may also lead to inherited breast cancers. However, these gene mutations are much rarer and do not increase the risk for breast cancer as much as the BRCA genes. They are not frequent causes of inherited breast cancer.

- **ATM:** The ATM gene normally helps repair damaged DNA. Inheriting 2 abnormal copies of this gene causes the disease ataxia-telangiectasia. Inheriting 1 mutated copy of this gene has been linked to a high rate of breast cancer in some families.

- **p53:** Inherited mutations of the p53 tumor suppressor gene cause the Li-Fraumeni syndrome (named after the 2 researchers who first described it). People with this syndrome are at increased risk for breast cancer, as well as several other types of cancer such as leukemia, brain tumors, and sarcomas (cancer of the bones or connective tissue). This is a rare cause of breast cancer.
- **CHEK2:** The Li-Fraumeni syndrome can also be caused by inherited mutations in the CHEK2 gene. Even when they do not cause this syndrome, inherited mutations of the CHEK2 gene increase breast cancer risk about twofold.
- **PTEN:** The PTEN gene normally helps regulate cell growth. Inherited mutations in this gene cause Cowden syndrome, a rare disorder in which people are at increased risk for both benign and malignant breast tumors, as well as growths in the digestive tract, thyroid, uterus, and ovaries.
- **CDH1:** Inherited mutations in the CDH1 gene cause hereditary diffuse gastric cancer, a syndrome in which people develop a rare type of stomach cancer at an early age. Women with mutations in this gene also are at increased risk for invasive lobular breast cancer.

Genetic testing can be done to look for mutations in the BRCA1 and BRCA2 genes (or, less commonly, in other genes such as PTEN or p53). Although testing may be helpful in some situations, the advantages and disadvantages should be considered carefully. For more information, see the section "Can Breast Cancer Be Prevented?" on page 37.

Family history of breast cancer

Breast cancer risk is higher among women whose close blood relatives have had the disease. Having one **first-degree relative** (mother, sister, or daughter) with breast cancer approximately doubles a woman's risk. Having 2 first-degree relatives increases the risk about threefold.

Although the exact risk is not known, women with a family history of breast cancer in a father or brother also are at increased risk for breast cancer. Altogether, less than 15% of women with breast cancer have had a family member with this disease. (Therefore, more than 85% of women who get breast cancer *do not* have a family history of this disease.)

Personal history of breast cancer

A woman with cancer in one breast has a three- to fourfold increased risk of a new cancer developing in the other breast or in another part of the same breast. This new cancer is different from a **recurrence** (return) of the first cancer.

Race and ethnicity

Breast cancer is slightly more likely to occur in white women than in black women. However, black women are more likely to die of breast cancer because they tend to have more aggressive tumors, although the reason for this is unknown. Asian, Hispanic, and Native American women have a lower risk of developing and dying of breast cancer.

Dense breast tissue

Women with denser breast tissue (as seen on a mammogram) are at higher risk for breast cancer. These women have more glandular tissue and less fatty tissue. Unfortunately, dense breast tissue can make it more difficult for doctors to spot problems on mammograms.

Certain benign breast conditions

Women who have certain benign breast conditions may be at increased risk for breast cancer. Some of these conditions are more closely linked to breast cancer risk than others. Doctors often divide benign breast conditions into the following 3 general groups, depending on how they affect risk.

Nonproliferative lesions: These conditions are not associated with overgrowth of breast tissue and do not seem to affect breast cancer risk. When risk is affected, it is to a very small extent.

These are the different types of **nonproliferative lesions**:

- fibrocystic disease (fibrosis and/or cysts)
- mild hyperplasia

- adenosis (non-sclerosing)
- ductal ectasia
- phyllodes tumor (benign)
- a single papilloma
- fat necrosis
- mastitis
- simple fibroadenoma
- other benign tumors (lipoma, hamartoma, hemangioma, and neurofibroma)

Proliferative lesions without atypia: These conditions show excessive growth of cells in the ducts or lobules of the breast tissue. They seem to raise a woman's risk for breast cancer slightly (1½ to 2 times the normal risk).

These are the different types of **proliferative lesions without atypia**:
- usual ductal hyperplasia (without atypia)
- complex fibroadenoma
- sclerosing adenosis
- several papillomas (or papillomatosis)
- radial scar

Proliferative lesions with atypia: In these conditions, there is excessive growth of cells in the ducts or lobules of the breast tissue, and the cells no longer appear normal. They have a stronger effect on breast cancer risk, raising it 4 to 5 times higher than normal.

These are the different types of **proliferative lesions with atypia**:
- atypical ductal hyperplasia (ADH)
- atypical lobular hyperplasia (ALH)

Women with a family history of breast cancer and either hyperplasia or atypical hyperplasia are at even higher risk for breast cancer.

For more information on these conditions, contact your American Cancer Society at **800-227-2345** and request the document *Non-cancerous Breast Conditions,* or visit our Web site, **cancer.org**.

Lobular carcinoma in situ

Women with lobular carcinoma in situ (LCIS) have a seven- to elevenfold increased risk for cancer to develop in either breast.

Menstrual periods

Women who have had more menstrual cycles because they started menstruating at an early age (before age 12) and/or went through **menopause** at a later age (after age 55) are at a slightly higher risk for breast cancer. This increased risk may be related to a higher lifetime exposure to the hormones estrogen and progesterone.

Previous chest radiation

Women who had radiation therapy to the chest area as treatment for another cancer (such as **Hodgkin disease** or **non-Hodgkin lymphoma**) as children or young adults are at significantly increased risk for breast cancer. This risk varies according to the patient's age at the time she underwent radiation therapy. If chemotherapy was also given, it may have stopped ovarian hormone production for some time, lowering the risk. The risk that breast cancer will develop as a result of chest radiation appears to be highest if the radiation was given during adolescence, when the breasts were still developing. Radiation treatment after age 40 does not seem to increase breast cancer risk.

Diethylstilbestrol exposure

From the 1940s through the 1960s, some pregnant women were given the drug **diethylstilbestrol (DES)** because it was believed to lower the chances of miscarriage. These women have a slightly increased risk of breast cancer. Women whose mothers took DES during pregnancy may also have a slightly higher risk of breast cancer. For more information on DES, contact your American Cancer Society at **800-227-2345** and request the document *DES Exposure: Questions and Answers,* or visit our Web site, **cancer.org**.

Lifestyle-Related Factors and Breast Cancer Risk

Reproductive history

Women who have had no pregnancies or who had their first child after age 30 have a slightly higher risk of getting breast cancer. Having many pregnancies and becoming pregnant at a young age reduce breast cancer risk. Pregnancy reduces a woman's total number of lifetime menstrual cycles, which may be the reason for this effect.

Recent oral contraceptive use

The risk of breast cancer is slightly higher in women using oral contraceptives (birth control pills) than in those who have never used them, but this risk seems to decline once the pills are stopped. Women who stopped using oral contraceptives more than 10 years ago do not appear to have any increased breast cancer risk. Women should discuss their other risk factors for breast cancer with their doctor when considering use of oral contraceptives.

Hormone therapy after menopause

Hormone therapy with estrogen (sometimes with progesterone) has been used for many years to help relieve symptoms of menopause and to help prevent osteoporosis (thinning of the bones). Earlier studies suggested that **postmenopausal hormone therapy (PHT)** might have other health benefits as well, but these benefits have not been found in more recent, better-designed studies. Other names for this therapy include **hormone replacement therapy (HRT)** and **menopausal hormone therapy (MHT)**.

There are 2 main types of hormone therapy. For women who still have a uterus (womb), doctors generally prescribe estrogen and progesterone (known as combined hormone therapy or HT). Because estrogen alone can increase the risk of uterine cancer, progesterone is added to help minimize this risk. For women who no longer have a uterus (those who have had a **hysterectomy**), estrogen alone can be prescribed. This is commonly known as **estrogen replacement therapy (ERT)** or just estrogen therapy (ET).

Combined HT: Use of combined hormone therapy after menopause increases the risk of breast cancer and may also increase the chances of dying of breast cancer. This increase in risk can be seen with as little as 2 years of use. Combined HT also increases the likelihood that the cancer may be found at a more advanced stage, possibly because it reduces the effectiveness of mammograms by increasing breast density. However, the increased risk from combined HT appears to apply only to current and recent users. A woman's risk of breast cancer seems to revert to that of the general population within 5 years of stopping combined treatment.

ERT: The use of estrogen alone after menopause does not appear to increase the risk of developing breast cancer significantly, if at all. However, some studies have shown that long-term use (for more than 10 years) of ERT does increase the risk of ovarian and breast cancer.

At this time, there appear to be few strong reasons to use postmenopausal hormone therapy (either combined HT or ERT), other than for short-term relief of menopausal symptoms. Along with the increased risk of breast cancer, combined HT also appears to increase the risk of heart disease, blood clots, and strokes. It does lower the risk of colorectal cancer and osteoporosis, but these benefits must be weighed against possible harm, especially since there are other effective ways to prevent and treat osteoporosis. Although ERT does not seem to have much effect on breast cancer risk, it does increase the risk of stroke. The increased risk associated with hormone therapy is the same for "bioidentical" and "natural" hormones as for synthetic hormones.

The decision to use HT after menopause should be made by a woman and her doctor after weighing the possible risks and benefits, based on the severity of her menopausal symptoms and her other risk factors for breast cancer, heart disease, and osteoporosis. If a woman and her doctor decide to try HT for symptoms of menopause, it is usually best to use it at the lowest dose needed to control symptoms and for as short a time as possible.

Breastfeeding

Some studies suggest that breastfeeding may slightly lower breast cancer risk, especially if breast-feeding is continued for 1½ to 2 years. But this has been a difficult area to study, especially in countries such as the United States, where breastfeeding for this long is uncommon. The explanation for this possible effect may be that breastfeeding reduces a woman's total number of lifetime menstrual cycles (similar to starting menstrual periods at a later age or going through early menopause).

Alcohol

Use of alcohol is clearly linked to an increased risk for breast cancer. The risk increases with the amount of alcohol consumed. Compared with non-drinkers, women who consume 1 alcoholic beverage a day have a very small increase in risk. Those who have 2 to 5 beverages daily have about 1½ times the risk of women who do not drink alcohol. Excessive alcohol use is also known to increase the risk of developing cancers of the mouth, throat, esophagus, and liver. The American Cancer Society recommends that women limit their consumption of alcohol to no more than one drink per day.

Being overweight or obese

Being overweight or obese has been found to increase breast cancer risk, especially for post-menopausal women. Before menopause, a woman's ovaries produce most of the body's estrogen, while fat tissue produces a small amount of estrogen. After menopause (when the ovaries stop making estrogen), most of a woman's estrogen comes from fat tissue. Having more fat tissue after menopause can increase your chance of getting breast cancer by raising estrogen levels. The connection between weight and breast cancer risk is complex, however. For example, the risk appears to increase for women who gain weight as adults but may not increase among women who have been overweight since childhood. Also, excess fat in the waist area may affect risk more than the same amount of fat in the hips and thighs. Researchers believe that fat cells in various parts of the body have subtle differences that may explain this risk.

The American Cancer Society recommends that women maintain a healthy weight throughout their lives by balancing food intake with physical activity and avoiding excessive weight gain.

Physical activity

Evidence is growing that physical activity in the form of exercise reduces breast cancer risk. The main question is this: How much exercise is needed to reduce risk? In one study from the Women's Health Initiative (WHI), as little as 1¼ to 2½ hours per week of brisk walking reduced a woman's risk by 18%. Walking 10 hours a week reduced the risk a little more. To reduce the risk of breast cancer, the American Cancer Society recommends 45 to 60 minutes of intentional physical activity 5 or more days a week.

Factors with Uncertain, Controversial, or Unproven Effects on Breast Cancer Risk

Diet and vitamin intake

Many studies have looked for a link between certain diets and breast cancer risk, but so far the results have been conflicting. Some studies have indicated that diet may play a role, whereas others found no evidence that diet influences breast cancer risk. In addition, no clear link to breast cancer was found in studies that examined the amount of fat in the diet, intake of fruits and vegetables, and intake of meat. Studies have also examined vitamin levels, again with inconsistent results. Some studies have shown an increased risk of breast cancer in women with higher levels of certain nutrients. But thus far, no study has shown that taking vitamins reduces breast cancer risk. This is not to say that there is no point in eating a healthy diet. A diet low in fat and high in fruits and vegetables may have other health benefits.

Most studies have found that breast cancer is less common in countries where the typical diet is low in total fat, polyunsaturated fat, and saturated fat. However, many studies of women in the United States have not found breast cancer risk to be related to dietary fat intake. Researchers are still not sure how to explain this apparent discrepancy.

It may be due, at least in part, to the effect of diet on body weight. Also, studies comparing diet and breast cancer risk in different countries are complicated by other differences (such as activity level, intake of other nutrients, and genetic factors) that might also alter breast cancer risk.

More research is needed to better understand the relationship between breast cancer risk and dietary fat. But it is clear that calories do count, and fat is a major source of calories. High-fat diets can lead to being overweight or obese, which is a risk factor for breast cancer. A diet high in fat also affects the risk for several other types of cancer, and intake of certain types of fat is clearly related to heart disease. The American Cancer Society recommends eating a healthy diet with an emphasis on plant sources. This includes eating 5 or more servings of vegetables and fruits each day, choosing whole grains over processed (refined) grains, and limiting consumption of processed and red meats.

Antiperspirants

Rumors circulating over the Internet have suggested that chemicals in underarm antiperspirants can be absorbed through the skin, interfere with lymph circulation, cause toxins to build up in the breast, and eventually lead to breast cancer. There is very little laboratory or population-based evidence to support this rumor. One small study has found trace levels of parabens (used as preservatives in antiperspirants and other products), which have weak estrogen-like properties, in a small sample of breast cancer tumors. However, the purpose of that study was not to determine whether parabens caused the tumors. That was a preliminary finding, and more research is needed to determine what effect, if any, parabens may have on breast cancer risk. Another large study of breast cancer causes found no increase in breast cancer in women who used underarm antiperspirants or shaved their underarms.

Bras

Another Internet rumor and at least one book have suggested that bras cause breast cancer by obstructing lymph flow. There is no solid scientific or clinical basis for this claim. Women who do not wear bras regularly may be more likely to be thinner or have less dense breasts, which could contribute to any perceived difference in risk.

Induced abortion

Several studies have provided very strong data that neither induced abortions nor spontaneous abortions (miscarriages) have an overall effect on the risk of breast cancer. For more detailed information, contact your American Cancer Society at **800-227-2345** and request the document *Is Abortion Linked to Breast Cancer?* or visit our Web site, **cancer.org**.

Breast implants

Several studies have found that breast implants do not increase breast cancer risk; however, silicone breast implants can cause scar tissue to form in the breast. Implants make it harder to see breast tissue on standard mammograms, but additional x-ray pictures called implant displacement views can be used to examine the breast tissue more thoroughly.

Chemicals in the environment

A great deal of research has been reported and more research is in progress to understand possible environmental influences on breast cancer risk. Of special interest are compounds in the environment that have been found in laboratory studies to have estrogen-like properties, which theoretically could affect breast cancer risk. For example, substances found in some plastics, certain cosmetics and personal care products, pesticides (such as DDE), and PCBs (polychlorinated biphenyls) seem to have such properties.

This issue understandably invokes a great deal of public concern, but research has not shown a clear link between breast cancer risk and exposure to these substances. Unfortunately, studying such effects in humans is difficult. More research is needed to better define the possible health effects of these and similar substances.

Tobacco smoke

Most studies have found no link between cigarette smoking and breast cancer. Although some studies have suggested that smoking increases the risk for breast cancer, this claim remains controversial.

An active focus of research is whether exposure to secondhand smoke increases the risk for breast cancer. Both first- and secondhand smoke contain chemicals that, in high concentrations, cause breast cancer in rodents. Chemicals in tobacco smoke reach breast tissue and can be found in breast milk. The evidence on secondhand smoke and breast cancer risk in human studies is not conclusive, at least in part because smokers have not been shown to be at increased risk. One possible explanation is that tobacco smoke may affect smokers differently from those who are just exposed to smoke.

A report from the California Environmental Protection Agency in 2005 concluded that the evidence about secondhand smoke and breast cancer is "consistent with a causal association" in younger, mostly premenopausal women. The 2006 U.S. Surgeon General's report, *The Health Consequences of Involuntary Exposure to Tobacco Smoke*, concluded that there is "suggestive but not sufficient" evidence of a link at this point. In any case, this possible link to breast cancer is yet another reason to avoid secondhand smoke.

Night work

Several studies have suggested that women who work at night—for example, nurses who work night shifts—may be at increased risk for breast cancer. This is a fairly recent finding, and more studies are looking at this issue. Some researchers think the effect may be due to changes in levels of melatonin, a hormone whose production is affected by the body's exposure to light, but other hormones are also being studied.

Do We Know What Causes Breast Cancer?

Although many risk factors may increase your chance of getting breast cancer, it is not known exactly how these risk factors cause cells to become cancerous. Hormones seem to play a role in many cases of breast cancer, but just how this happens is not completely understood.

Certain changes in DNA can cause normal breast cells to become cancerous. DNA is the chemical in each cell that makes up our genes—the instructions for how our cells should function. For example, we usually resemble our parents because they are the source of our DNA. However, DNA affects more than how a person looks. Some genes contain instructions for controlling when our cells grow, divide, and die. Certain genes that speed up cell division are called **oncogenes**. Others that slow down cell division, or cause cells to die at the right time, are called **tumor suppressor genes**. Different types of cancer can be caused by DNA mutations that "turn on" oncogenes or "turn off" tumor suppressor genes.

Inherited Gene Mutations

Certain inherited DNA changes can increase the risk for cancer and are responsible for the cancers that run in some families. For example, the BRCA genes (BRCA1 and BRCA2) are tumor suppressor genes. Mutations in these genes can be inherited from parents. When they are mutated, they no longer suppress abnormal growth, and cancer is more likely to develop.

Women have already begun to benefit from advances in the understanding of how genetics affects breast cancer risk. Genetic testing can identify some women who have inherited mutations in the BRCA1 or BRCA2 tumor suppressor genes (or—less commonly—in other genes, such as p53 or PTEN). These women can then take steps to reduce the risk that breast cancer will develop and to monitor changes in their breasts carefully to find cancer at an earlier, more treatable stage. These steps will be discussed in more detail in later sections of this book.

Acquired Gene Mutations

Most DNA mutations related to breast cancer occur in breast cells during a woman's life rather than having been inherited. These acquired mutations of oncogenes and/or tumor suppressor genes may result from such factors as radiation or cancer-causing chemicals. But so far, the causes of most acquired mutations that may lead to breast cancer remain unknown. Most breast cancers have several gene mutations that are acquired. Tests that detect acquired gene changes may help doctors more accurately predict the prognosis for some women with breast cancer. For example, tests can identify women whose breast cancer cells have too many copies of the HER2 oncogene. These cancers tend to be more aggressive; however, drugs have been developed that specifically target cancers with too many copies of HER2.

Prevention and Detection

Can Breast Cancer Be Prevented?

There is no sure way to prevent breast cancer. But there are steps all women can take to reduce their risk and help increase the odds of detecting cancer at an early, more treatable stage.

Lowering Your Risk

You can lower your risk of breast cancer by changing those risk factors that can be changed (see the section, "What Are the Risk Factors for Breast Cancer?" on pages 17–34). Women who limit alcohol intake, exercise regularly, and maintain a healthy body weight have a lower risk of breast cancer. Women who choose to breastfeed for at least several months may also get an added benefit of reducing their breast cancer risk. You can also avoid raising your risk by not using hormone therapy after menopause.

Whether environmental chemicals that have estrogen-like properties (such as those found in some plastic bottles or certain cosmetics and personal care products) increase breast cancer risk is not clear at this time. If there is an increased risk, it is likely to be very small. Still, women who are concerned may choose to avoid products that contain these substances when possible.

Finding Breast Cancer Early

Other than lifestyle changes, the most important action a woman can take is to follow early detection guidelines. Following the American Cancer Society's recommendations for early detection (see page 45) will not prevent breast cancer, but it can make it more likely that any cancer will be detected when the likelihood of successful treatment is greatest.

For Women Who Are or May Be at Increased Risk

If you are a woman at increased risk for breast cancer (for example, because you have a strong family history of breast cancer, a known genetic mutation of a BRCA gene, or you have had DCIS, LCIS, or biopsies that have shown precancerous changes), there are ways to reduce your chances of getting breast cancer. Before deciding which, if any, of the following steps may be right for you, talk with your doctor to understand more about your risk and to what extent these approaches will lower it.

Genetic testing for BRCA gene mutations

Although many women may have relatives with breast cancer, in most cases this is not the result of BRCA gene mutations. Genetic testing for these mutations can be expensive and the results are often not clear-cut. Testing can have a wide range of consequences that need to be considered.

Testing should only be done when there is a reasonable suspicion that a mutation may be present.

The U.S. Preventive Services Task Force (USPSTF) recommends that only women with a strong family history be considered for genetic testing for BRCA mutations. This group represents only about 2% of adult women in the United States. The USPSTF recommends that women who are not of Ashkenazi (Eastern European) Jewish heritage be referred for genetic evaluation if they have any of the following:

- 2 first-degree relatives (mother, sisters, or daughters) with breast cancer, at least one of whom was younger than 50 at diagnosis
- 3 or more first- or second-degree relatives (mothers, sisters, daughters, grandmothers, or aunts) with breast cancer
- incidences of both breast and ovarian cancer among first- or second-degree relatives
- a first-degree relative with cancer in both breasts
- 2 or more first- or second-degree relatives with ovarian cancer
- a male relative with breast cancer

Women of Ashkenazi (Eastern European) Jewish heritage should be referred for genetic evaluation if they have any of the following:

- a first-degree relative with breast or ovarian cancer
- 2 second-degree relatives on the same side of the family with breast or ovarian cancer

If you are considering genetic testing, you should first talk to a genetic counselor, nurse, or doctor who is qualified to explain and interpret the results of these tests. It is very important to understand what genetic testing can and cannot tell you and to then carefully weigh the benefits and risks of testing before proceeding. Testing is expensive and may not be covered by health insurance. For more information, call your American Cancer Society at **800-227-2345** and request the document *Genetic Testing: What You Need to Know*, or visit our Web site, **cancer.org**. You may also want to visit the National Cancer Institute Web site (www.cancer.gov/cancertopics/Genetic-Testing -for-Breast-and-Ovarian-Cancer-Risk).

Breast cancer chemoprevention

Chemoprevention is the use of drugs to reduce the risk of cancer. Several drugs have been studied for use in lowering breast cancer risk.

Tamoxifen: Tamoxifen (Nolvadex) is a drug that blocks some of the effects of estrogen on breast tissue. It has been used for many years to reduce the risk of recurrence in localized breast cancer and as a treatment for advanced breast cancer when the tumor is estrogen receptor–positive (see the section "How Is Breast Cancer Treated?" on pages 109–172). Several studies have found that tamoxifen can also lower the risk for breast cancer in women who are at increased risk for the disease.

Results from the Breast Cancer Prevention Trial (BCPT) have shown that women at increased risk for breast cancer are less likely to get the disease if they take tamoxifen. Women enrolled in this study took either tamoxifen or a placebo pill for 5 years. After 7 years of follow-up, women taking tamoxifen had 42% fewer breast cancers than women who took the placebo, although there was no difference in the risk of dying of breast cancer. Tamoxifen is approved for reducing breast cancer risk in women at high risk.

Because tamoxifen has side effects that include increased risk of endometrial (uterine) cancer and blood clots, women should consider the possible benefits and risks of tamoxifen before deciding whether it is right for them.

Whereas it appears that tamoxifen reduces breast cancer risk in women with BRCA2 gene mutations, the same may not be true for those with BRCA1 mutations.

Raloxifene: Like tamoxifen, raloxifene also blocks the effect of estrogen on breast tissue. A study comparing the effectiveness of the 2 drugs in women after menopause, called the Study of Tamoxifen and Raloxifene (STAR) trial, found that raloxifene worked nearly as well as tamoxifen in reducing the risk of invasive breast cancer and noninvasive cancer (DCIS or LCIS). Raloxifene also was associated with lower risks of certain side effects such as uterine cancer and blood clots in the legs or lungs, compared with tamoxifen (although the risk of blood clots was still higher than normal). Raloxifene is approved to reduce breast cancer risk in postmenopausal women who have osteoporosis (bone thinning) or who are at high risk for breast cancer.

Aromatase inhibitors: Drugs such as anastrozole (Arimidex), letrozole (Femara), and exemestane (Aromasin) are also being studied as breast cancer chemopreventive agents in postmenopausal women. **Aromatase inhibitors** are already being used to help prevent breast cancer recurrences. They work by blocking production of the small amounts of estrogen that postmenopausal women normally make. However, they can also have side effects, including joint pain and stiffness and bone loss, leading to a higher risk of osteoporosis. These drugs have not been approved for reducing the risk of developing breast cancer at this time.

Other drugs: Studies are under way to examine the effects of other drugs on breast cancer risk. For example, some studies have found that women who take aspirin or **nonsteroidal antiinflammatory drugs (NSAIDs)** such as ibuprofen appear to have a lower risk of breast cancer. NSAIDs and several other drugs and dietary supplements are being studied to determine whether they can lower breast cancer risk, although none are approved for reducing breast cancer risk at this time.

You can find more information on these drugs in the section "How Is Breast Cancer Treated?" on pages 151–155. For more information on the possible benefits and risks of chemopreventive drugs, contact your American Cancer Society at **800-227-2345** and request the document *Medicines to Reduce Breast Cancer Risk*, or visit our Web site, **cancer.org**.

Prophylactic (preventive) surgery

For the few women who are at very high risk for breast cancer, prophylactic (preventive) surgery to remove the breasts or ovaries may be an option.

Prophylactic bilateral mastectomy: Removing both breasts before cancer is diagnosed can reduce the risk of breast cancer by up to 97%. Some women who receive a diagnosis of cancer in one breast may choose to have the other healthy breast removed as well, to prevent a second breast cancer diagnosis. Breast removal cannot completely prevent breast cancer because even the most careful surgeon will leave behind at least a few breast cells, which could eventually become cancerous. These are some of the reasons for considering prophylactic surgery:

- mutated BRCA genes found by genetic testing
- previous cancer in one breast
- strong family history (breast cancer in several close relatives)
- biopsy specimens showing lobular carcinoma in situ (LCIS)

There is no way to know ahead of time whether prophylactic bilateral mastectomy will benefit every patient. For some women with BRCA mutations, breast cancer will develop early in life, and they will have a high risk of getting a second breast cancer. A prophylactic mastectomy before cancer occurs might add many years to their lives. Even though most women with BRCA mutations get breast cancer, some do not. These women would not benefit from the surgery and would still have to deal with its after-effects.

Second opinions are strongly recommended before any woman decides to have this surgery. The American Cancer Society Board of Directors has stated that "only very strong clinical and/or pathologic indications warrant doing this type of preventive operation." Nonetheless, after careful consideration, prophylactic bilateral mastectomy might be the right choice for some women at high risk for breast cancer.

Prophylactic oophorectomy: Women with a BRCA mutation may reduce their risk of breast cancer by 50% or more by having their ovaries surgically removed before menopause. Removing the ovaries decreases a woman's breast cancer risk because the surgery removes the body's main sources of estrogen. This procedure is called prophylactic oophorectomy. In addition to increased breast cancer risk, women with a BRCA mutation should understand that they are also at high risk for ovarian cancer. Most doctors recommend that women with BRCA mutations have their ovaries surgically removed after their childbearing years to lower risk.

Can Breast Cancer Be Found Early?

Screening refers to tests and examinations used to find a disease in people who do not have any symptoms. The goal of screening examinations, such as mammograms, is to find cancer before any symptoms begin. Breast cancers that are found because they can be felt tend to be larger and are more likely to have already spread beyond the breast. In contrast, breast cancers detected during screening examinations are more likely to be small and still confined to the breast. The size of a breast cancer and how far it has spread are important factors in predicting the prognosis for a woman with breast cancer.

Most doctors agree that early detection tests for breast cancer save thousands of lives each year, and that many more lives could be saved if more women and their health care providers took advantage of these tests. Following the American Cancer Society's guidelines for the early detection of breast cancer improves the chances that breast cancer can be diagnosed at an early stage and treated successfully.

American Cancer Society Recommendations for Early Breast Cancer Detection

Women age 40 and older should have a screening mammogram every year and should continue to do so for as long as they are in good health.

- Current evidence in support of mammograms is even stronger than in the past. In particular, recent evidence has confirmed that mammograms offer substantial benefit for women in their 40s. Women can feel confident about the benefits associated with regular mammograms for finding cancer early. However, mammograms also have limitations. A mammogram will miss some cancers, and it will detect abnormalities that are found after biopsy to be benign.

- Women should be told about the benefits, limitations, and potential harms linked with regular screening. Mammograms can miss some cancers. But despite their limitations, they remain a very effective and valuable tool for decreasing suffering and death from breast cancer.

- Mammograms for older women should be based on the individual, her health, and other serious illnesses, such as congestive heart failure, end-stage renal disease, chronic obstructive pulmonary disease, and moderate-to-severe dementia. Age alone should not be the reason to stop having regular mammograms. As long as a woman is in good health and would be a candidate for treatment, she should continue to have screening mammograms.

Women in their 20s and 30s should have a clinical breast examination (CBE) as part of a periodic (regular) health examination by a health care professional, at least every 3 years. After the age of 40, women should have a CBE by a health care professional every year.

- A clinical breast examination (CBE) is a complement to mammograms and gives women an opportunity to discuss changes in their breasts with their doctor or nurse. Early detection testing and factors in their medical or personal history that might affect breast cancer risk should also be discussed.

- There may be some benefit in having the CBE shortly before the mammogram because women can receive instructions during the examination about how to become more familiar with their own breasts. Women should also be given information about the benefits and limitations of CBE and breast self-examination (BSE). Breast cancer risk is very low for women in their 20s and gradually increases with age. Women should be told to promptly report any new breast symptoms to a health professional.

Breast self-examination (BSE) is an option for women starting in their 20s. Women should be told about the benefits and limitations of BSE and should report any changes to their health care professional right away.

- Doing BSE regularly is one way for women to know how their breasts normally look and feel and to notice any changes. Research has shown that BSE plays a small role in detecting breast cancer compared with finding a breast lump by chance. Some women prefer to do BSE on a regular schedule (usually monthly after their period), which involves a systematic step-by-step examination of the look and feel of their breasts. Just after a woman's period, the breasts are less tender and can tolerate a thorough examination. Other women are more comfortable simply looking at and feeling their breasts in a less systematic way, such as while showering or getting dressed, or doing an occasional thorough exam. The goal, with or without BSE, is to report any breast changes to a doctor or nurse right away.

- If you choose to do BSE, have your technique reviewed by your doctor or nurse during your physical examination. Women can sometimes be so concerned about "doing it right" that they become stressed about the technique. Some women choose not to do BSE or not to follow a regular schedule; however, it is in your best interest to consider the benefits of BSE. By performing breast self-examinations regularly, you will get to know how your breasts normally look and feel. You will also be able to more readily detect any changes, such as a lump or swelling, skin irritation or **dimpling**, nipple pain or retraction (turning inward), redness or scaliness of the nipple or breast skin, or a discharge other than breast milk. If you notice any changes, see your health care provider as soon as possible for evaluation. Remember that most of the time, however, these breast changes are not cancer-related.

Women at high risk (greater than 20% lifetime risk) should undergo magnetic resonance imaging (MRI) and a screening mammogram every

year. **Women at moderately increased risk (15% to 20% lifetime risk) should talk with their doctors about the benefits and limitations of adding MRI screening to their yearly mammogram. Yearly MRI screening is not recommended for women whose lifetime risk of breast cancer is less than 15%.**

- Women at high risk include those who have one or more of the following characteristics:
  ○ a known BRCA1 or BRCA2 gene mutation
  ○ a first-degree relative (parent, brother, sister, or child) with a BRCA1 or BRCA2 gene mutation, but they have not had genetic testing themselves
  ○ a lifetime risk of breast cancer of 20% to 25% or greater, according to risk assessment tools that are based mainly on family history (as with the Claus model, see next page)
  ○ radiation therapy to the chest when they were between the ages of 10 and 30
  ○ Li-Fraumeni syndrome, Cowden syndrome, or hereditary diffuse gastric cancer, or a first-degree relative with one of these syndromes
- Women at moderately increased risk include those who have one or more of the following characteristics:
  ○ a lifetime risk of breast cancer of 15% to 20%, according to risk assessment tools that are based mainly on family history

- - a personal history of breast cancer, ductal carcinoma in situ (DCIS), lobular carcinoma in situ (LCIS), atypical ductal hyperplasia (ADH), or atypical lobular hyperplasia (ALH)
  - extremely dense breasts or unevenly dense breasts when viewed by mammograms
- If an MRI is used, it should be in addition to, not instead of, a screening mammogram. While an MRI is a more sensitive test (meaning it is more likely to detect cancer than a mammogram), it may still miss some cancers that a mammogram would detect.
- For most women at high risk, screening with MRI and mammograms should begin at the age of 30 and continue for as long as a woman is in good health. Because evidence is limited regarding the best age at which to start screening, this decision should be made with the counsel of the woman's health care provider, taking into account her personal circumstances and preferences.
- Several risk assessment tools, with names such as the Gail model, the Claus model, and the Tyrer-Cuzick model, are available to help health care professionals estimate a woman's breast cancer risk. These tools are based mainly on family history and give approximate, rather than precise,

estimates of breast cancer risk based on different combinations of risk factors and different data sets. As a result, they may give different risk estimates for the same woman. For example, the Gail model bases its risk estimates on certain personal risk factors, such as age at start of menstruation and history of prior breast biopsies, along with any history of breast cancer in first-degree relatives. The Claus model bases its risk estimate on family history of breast cancer in both first- and second-degree relatives. Using the same data, these 2 models could easily give different estimates. Therefore, the results of these risk assessment tools should be discussed by a woman and her doctor when they are being used in determining whether to start MRI screening.

- Women who start MRI screening should do so at a facility that can perform an MRI–guided breast biopsy at the same time if needed. Otherwise, you will have to have a second MRI at another facility at the time of biopsy.
- There is no evidence at this time that MRI is an effective screening tool for women at average risk. While MRIs are more sensitive than mammograms, they also have a higher false-positive rate (meaning it is more likely to find an abnormality that is not cancer), which would result in unneeded biopsies and other tests.

The American Cancer Society believes that a combined approach to early detection is clearly better than any one exam or test alone. The use of mammograms, MRI (in women at high risk), clinical breast exams, and awareness of any changes in the breast offers women the best chance to reduce their risk of dying of breast cancer. Without question, a clinical breast examination without a mammogram would not detect many breast cancers that are too small to be felt manually but can be seen on mammograms. Although mammograms are a sensitive screening method, a small percentage of breast cancers are not detected on mammograms but can be felt by a woman or her doctors. For women at high risk of breast cancer, such as those with BRCA gene mutations or a strong family history, both an MRI and a mammogram are recommended.

Mammograms

A mammogram is an **x-ray** of the breast. A diagnostic mammogram is used to diagnose breast disease in women who have breast symptoms or an abnormal result on a screening mammogram. Screening mammograms are used to look for breast disease in women who are asymptomatic; that is, they appear to have no breast problems. Screening mammograms usually take 2 views (x-ray pictures taken from different angles) of each breast. For some patients, such as women with breast implants, more pictures may be needed to include as much breast tissue as possible. Women who are breastfeeding can still get mammograms, although the mammogram will probably not be quite as accurate because the breast tissue tends to be dense.

Although breast x-rays have been done for more than 70 years, the modern mammogram has only existed since 1969. That was the first year x-ray units specifically for breast imaging were available. Modern mammography equipment uses very low levels of radiation, usually a dose of about 0.1 to 0.2 rads per picture (a rad is a measure of radiation dose). Strict guidelines ensure that mammogram equipment is safe and uses the lowest dose of radiation possible. Many people are concerned about the exposure to x-rays, but the level of radiation used in modern mammograms does not significantly increase the risk for breast cancer. To put this into perspective, consider this example: If a woman has yearly mammograms from the age of 40 to 90, she will receive between 20 and 40 rads. If a woman with breast cancer is treated with radiation, she will receive approximately 5,000 rads.

For a mammogram, the breast is pressed between 2 plates to flatten and spread the tissue. Although this may be uncomfortable for a moment, it is necessary to produce a good, "readable" mammogram. The compression lasts only a few seconds. The entire procedure for a screening mammogram takes about 20 minutes. The mammogram produces a black and white image of the breast tissue (either on a large sheet of film or as a digital computer image) that is read, or interpreted, by a radiologist (a doctor trained to interpret images from x-rays, ultrasound, MRI, and related tests).

Some advances in technology, such as digital mammography, may help doctors read mammograms more accurately. They are described in the section "How Is Breast Cancer Diagnosed?" on pages 69–90.

What the doctor looks for on your mammogram

The doctor reading the films will look for several types of changes.

Calcifications are tiny mineral deposits within the breast tissue, which look like small white spots on the films. They may or may not be caused by cancer. There are 2 types of calcifications:

- **Macrocalcifications** are coarse (larger) calcium deposits and are most likely caused by aging of the breast arteries, old injuries, or inflammation. These deposits are related to noncancerous conditions and do not require biopsy. Macrocalcifications are found in about half of women over 50, and in about 1 of 10 women under the age of 50.
- **Microcalcifications** are tiny specks of calcium in the breast. They may appear alone or in clusters. Microcalcifications seen on a mammogram are more of a cause for concern, but they usually do not mean that cancer is present. The shape and layout of microcalcifications help the radiologist judge how likely it is that cancer is present. If the calcifications look suspicious, a biopsy will be performed.

A **mass**, which may occur with or without calcifications, is another important change that can be seen on mammograms. Masses can be many things, including cysts (noncancerous, fluid-filled sacs) and noncancerous solid tumors (such as fibroadenomas). They may also be cancerous and usually should be biopsied if they are not cysts.

- A cyst and a tumor can feel alike on a physical exam and can also look the same on a mammogram. To confirm that a mass is really a cyst, either a breast ultrasound or the removal (aspiration) of fluid from the cyst with a thin, hollow needle is needed.

- If a mass is not a simple cyst (if it is at least partly solid), you may need to have more **imaging tests**. Some masses can be monitored with periodic mammograms, whereas others may need a biopsy. The size, shape, and margins (edges) of the mass help the radiologist determine whether cancer is present.

It is very important that you give your radiologist copies of your previous mammograms. They can show that a mass or calcification has not changed for many years. This would mean that it is probably a benign condition and a biopsy is not needed.

Limitations of mammograms

A mammogram cannot prove that an abnormal area is cancerous. To confirm whether cancer is present, a small amount of tissue must be removed and examined under a microscope, a procedure known as a biopsy. Biopsy is described in more detail in the section "How Is Breast Cancer Diagnosed?" on pages 79–83.

You should also be aware that mammograms do not always reveal breast cancer. If you have a breast lump, you should have it checked by your doctor and consider having a biopsy even if your mammogram result is normal.

For some women, such as those with breast implants, additional pictures may be needed. Breast implants make it harder to see breast tissue on standard mammograms, but additional x-ray pictures with implant displacement and compression views can be used to more completely examine the breast tissue.

Mammograms are not perfect. They do not work as well in younger women because a younger woman's breasts are often dense, which can hide a tumor. Pregnant women and women who are breastfeeding may also have dense breast tissue. Since most breast cancer occurs in older women (in whom breast tissue is not as dense), problems caused by density are usually not a major concern. However, this limitation can be a problem for young women who are at high risk for breast cancer (because of gene mutations, a strong family history of breast cancer, or other factors) because they often get breast cancer at a younger age. For this reason, the American Cancer Society now recommends MRI scans in addition to mammograms for screening in women at high risk.

For more information on imaging tests, also see the section "How Is Breast Cancer Diagnosed?" on pages 71–77. You can also call your American Cancer Society at **800-227-2345** and request the document *Mammograms and Other Breast Imaging Procedures,* or visit our Web site, **cancer.org**.

What to expect when you have a mammogram

- To have a mammogram, you must undress above the waist. The staff at the facility will give you a wrap to wear.
- A technologist will be there to position your breasts for the mammogram. Most technologists are women. You and the technologist are the only ones in the room during the mammogram.
- To get a high-quality mammogram picture with excellent image quality, it is necessary to flatten the breast slightly. The technologist places the breast on the lower plate of the mammogram machine, which is made of metal and has a drawer to hold the x-ray film or the camera to produce a digital image. The upper plate is made of plastic and is lowered to compress the breast for a few seconds while the technologist takes a picture.
- The whole procedure takes about 20 minutes. The actual breast compression only lasts a few seconds.
- You will feel some discomfort when your breasts are compressed. For some women, compression can be painful. Try not to schedule a mammogram when your breasts are likely to be tender, such as the time just before or during your period.

- All mammogram facilities are now required to send your results to you within 30 days. Generally, you will be contacted within 5 working days if there is a problem with the mammogram.
- Only 2 to 4 mammograms of every 1,000 lead to a diagnosis of cancer. About 10% of women who have a mammogram will require more tests, and the majority will only need an additional mammogram. Do not panic if you require more tests. Only 8% to 10% of those women will need a biopsy, and most (80%) of those biopsies will not be cancerous.

If you are a woman aged 40 or older, you should get a mammogram every year. You can schedule the next one while you are at the facility and/or request a reminder.

Tips for having a mammogram

Here are some useful suggestions for making sure that you receive a quality mammogram:

- If it is not posted visibly near the receptionist's desk, ask to see the **U.S. Food and Drug Administration (FDA)** certificate that is issued to all facilities that offer mammography. The FDA requires that all facilities meet high professional standards of safety and quality in order to be a provider of mammography services. A facility may not provide mammography without certification.

- Use a facility that either specializes in mammography or does many mammograms a day.
- If you are satisfied that the facility is of high quality, continue to go there on a regular basis so that your mammograms can be compared from year to year.
- If you are going to a facility for the first time, bring a list of the places and the dates of mammograms, biopsies, or other breast treatments you have had in the past.
- If you have had mammograms at another facility, try to obtain copies of those mammograms and bring them with you to the new facility (or have them sent there) so that they can be compared with the new ones.
- On the day of the mammogram, do not wear deodorant or antiperspirant. Some of these products contain substances that can interfere with the reading of the mammogram by appearing on the x-ray film as white spots.
- You may find it more convenient to wear a skirt or pants (rather than a dress, for example), so that you only need to remove your blouse for the mammogram.
- Schedule your mammogram when your breasts are not tender or swollen to help reduce discomfort and to ensure a good picture. Try to avoid scheduling your mammogram for the week before your period.

- Always describe any breast symptoms or problems you are having to the technologist who is doing the mammogram. Be prepared to describe any medical history that could affect your breast cancer risk— such as surgery, hormone use, or family or personal history of breast cancer. Discuss any new findings or problems in your breasts with your doctor or nurse before having a mammogram.
- If you do not hear from your doctor within 10 days, do not assume that your mammogram was normal—call your doctor or the facility.

Help with mammogram costs

Medicare, Medicaid, and most private health insurance plans cover mammogram costs or a percentage of them. Low-cost mammograms are available in most communities. For information about facilities in your area, contact your American Cancer Society at **800-227-2345** or visit our Web site, **cancer.org**.

Breast cancer screening is now more available to medically underserved women through the National Breast and Cervical Cancer Early Detection Program (NBCCEDP). This program helps low-income, uninsured, and underinsured women gain access to breast and cervical cancer screening and diagnostic services. Currently the NBCCEDP funds all 50 states, the District of Columbia, 5 U.S. territories, and 12 American Indian/Alaska Native tribes or tribal organizations. Although the program is administered within each state, the Centers for Disease Control and Prevention (CDC) provides matching funds and support to each state program. Each state's Department of Health has information on how to contact the nearest program. The program is only designed to provide screening. But if cancer is discovered, the program will cover further diagnostic testing and a surgical consultation.

The Breast and Cervical Cancer Prevention and Treatment Act, passed in 2000, provides the option to offer women in the NBCCEDP access to treatment through Medicaid. This program helps women focus their energies on fighting their disease, instead of worrying about how to pay for treatment. All states and the District of Columbia participate in this program.

To learn more about these programs, please contact the CDC at 800-CDC INFO (800-232-4636) or online at www.cdc.gov/cancer/nbccedp.

Clinical Breast Examination

A **clinical breast examination (CBE)** is an examination of your breasts by a health care professional, such as a doctor, nurse practitioner, nurse, or physician assistant. For this exam, you will need to undress from the waist up. Your health care professional will first look at your breasts for abnormalities in size or shape or changes in the skin of the breasts or nipple. Then, using the pads of the fingers, the examiner will gently palpate (feel) your breasts. Special attention will be given to the shape and texture of the breasts, the location of any lumps, and whether such lumps are attached to the skin or to deeper tissues. The area under both arms will also be examined.

The CBE is a good opportunity for women who do not know how to examine their breasts to learn the proper technique from their health care professionals. Ask your doctor or nurse to teach you and to watch your technique.

Breast Awareness and Self-examination

Beginning in their 20s, women should be told about the benefits and limitations of **breast self-examination (BSE)**. Women should know how their breasts normally look and feel and report any changes in their breasts to a health professional as soon as they are found. Finding a change in the breast does not necessarily mean there is cancer.

You can notice changes by being aware of how your breasts normally look and feel and by feeling your breasts for changes (breast awareness). You can also choose to use a step-by-step approach (discussed next) and use a specific schedule to examine your breasts.

If you choose to do BSE, the information provided next is a step-by-step approach for the examination. The best time to examine your breasts is when they are not tender or swollen (as they are likely to be in the week just before your period). Women who examine their breasts should have their technique reviewed during their periodic health examinations by their health care professional.

Women with breast implants can do BSE, too. It may be helpful to have the surgeon help identify the edges of the implant so that you know what you are feeling. Some health care professionals believe that the implants "push out" the breast tissue and may actually make it easier to examine. Women who are pregnant or breastfeeding can also examine their breasts regularly.

It is acceptable for women to choose not to do BSE or to do BSE once in a while. Women who choose not to do BSE should still be aware of the normal look and feel of their breasts and report any changes to their doctor right away.

How to examine your breasts

- Lie down and place your right arm behind your head. This first part of the breast self-examination is done lying down, not standing up. This is because the breast tissue spreads evenly over the chest wall and is thinnest when you are lying down, making it much easier to feel all the breast tissue.
- Use the finger pads of the 3 middle fingers on your left hand to feel for lumps in the

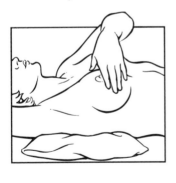
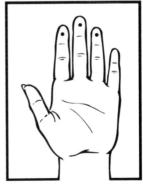

right breast. Use overlapping dime-sized circular motions of the finger pads to feel the breast tissue.

- Use 3 different levels of pressure to feel all the breast tissue. Light pressure is needed to feel the tissue closest to the skin; medium pressure to feel a little deeper; and firm pressure to feel the tissue closest to the chest and ribs. It is normal to feel a firm ridge in the lower curve of each breast, but you should tell your doctor if you feel anything else out of the ordinary. If you are not sure how hard to press, talk with your doctor or nurse. Feel each area of breast tissue with all 3 pressure levels before moving on to the next spot.

- Starting at an imaginary line drawn straight down from your underarm, move across the breast in an up-and-down pattern, moving across the breast to the middle of the sternum or breastbone. Be sure to check the entire breast area by going down until you feel only ribs and up to the neck or clavicle (collarbone).

- There is some evidence to suggest that the up-and-down pattern (sometimes called the vertical pattern) is the most effective pattern for covering the entire breast without missing any breast tissue.

- Repeat the examination on your left breast, putting your left arm behind your head and using the finger pads of your right hand to do the examination.

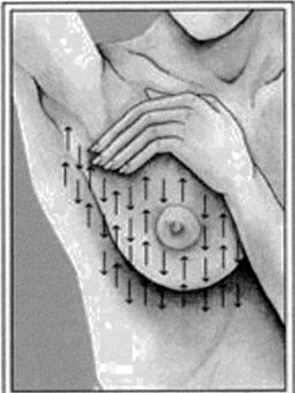

Breast Self-Examination

Examine up to the collarbone,
out to underarm, in to middle of chest,
and down to bottom of rib cage

- Next, while standing in front of a mirror with your hands pressing firmly down on your hips, look at your breasts for any changes in size, shape, contour, dimpling, or for any redness or scaliness of the nipple or breast skin. (Pressing down on the hips contracts the chest wall muscles and enhances any breast changes.)
- Examine each underarm while sitting up or standing and with your arm only slightly raised so you can easily feel in this area. Raising your arm straight up tightens the tissue in this area and makes it harder to examine.

This procedure for doing breast self-examination is different from previous recommendations. These changes represent an extensive review of the medical literature and input from an expert advisory group. There is evidence that the lying-down position, the examination area, the pattern of coverage of the breast, and the use of different amounts of pressure increase a woman's ability to find abnormalities.

Magnetic Resonance Imaging

As discussed previously, **magnetic resonance imaging (MRI)** is recommended, along with a yearly mammogram, for certain women at high risk for breast cancer. MRI is not generally recommended as a screening tool by itself. Although it is a sensitive test, it may still miss some cancers that mammograms would detect.

MRI scans use magnets and radio waves (instead of x-rays) to produce very detailed, cross-sectional images of the body. To be most useful, the MRI for breast imaging should be performed using a contrast material (**gadolinium**) that is injected into a vein in the arm before or during the examination. This improves the ability of the MRI to clearly show breast tissue details. (For more details on how the MRI is done, see the section, "How Is Breast Cancer Diagnosed?" on pages 74–75.)

Although an MRI is more sensitive than a mammogram in detecting cancers, it also has a higher false-positive rate (where the test finds an abnormality that is not cancer), which results in increased biopsies. This is why MRI is not recommended as a screening test for women at average risk of breast cancer, as it would result in unneeded biopsies and other tests in a large portion of these women.

Just as mammography uses x-ray machines that are specially designed for the breasts, a breast MRI also requires special equipment. Breast MRI machines produce higher-quality images than MRI machines that are designed for head, chest, or abdominal scanning. However, many hospitals and imaging centers do not have dedicated breast MRI equipment available. It is important that screening MRIs be done at facilities that can perform MRI–guided breast biopsies. Otherwise, the MRI will need to be repeated at another facility if a biopsy is needed.

MRI scans are more expensive than mammography. Most major insurance companies will likely pay for these screening tests if a woman can be shown to be at high risk, but it is not yet clear whether all insurers will do so. At this time, there are concerns about the costs of and limited access to high-quality MRI breast screening services for women at high risk for breast cancer.

Diagnosis and Staging

How Is Breast Cancer Diagnosed?

Although breast cancer is sometimes found after symptoms appear, many women with early-stage breast cancer have no symptoms. This is why getting the recommended screening tests (as described in the previous chapter) before symptoms develop is so important.

If something suspicious is found during a screening examination, or if you have any of the symptoms of breast cancer described on page 70, your doctor will use one or more methods to determine whether the disease is present. If cancer is found, other tests will be done to determine the stage (extent) of the cancer.

Although widespread use of screening mammograms has increased the number of breast cancers found before they cause symptoms, some breast cancers are not found by mammogram, either because the test was not done or because, even under ideal conditions, mammograms do not find every breast cancer.

Signs and Symptoms of Breast Cancer

The most common sign of breast cancer is a new lump or mass. A painless, hard mass that has irregular edges is more likely to be cancerous, but breast cancers can be tender, soft, or rounded. For this reason, it is important that any new breast mass or lump be checked by a health care professional experienced in diagnosing breast diseases.

These are other possible signs of breast cancer:

- swelling of all or part of the breast (even if no distinct lump is felt)
- skin irritation or dimpling
- breast or nipple pain
- **nipple retraction** (turning inward)
- redness, scaliness, or thickening of the nipple or breast skin
- a discharge other than breast milk

Sometimes breast cancer can spread to axillary lymph nodes (those under the arm) and cause a lump or swelling even before the original tumor in the breast is large enough to be felt.

Medical History and Physical Examination

If you have any symptoms that might be due to breast cancer, see your doctor as soon as possible. Your doctor will ask questions about your symptoms, any other health problems, and possible risk factors for benign breast conditions or breast cancer.

Your breasts will be thoroughly examined for any lumps or suspicious areas. Your doctor will palpate (feel) any suspicious areas to determine their texture, size, and relationship to the skin and chest muscles. Any changes in the nipples or the skin of your breasts will also be noted. The doctor may feel the lymph nodes in the underarm and above the collarbones. If the lymph nodes are enlarged or firm, this could indicate that cancer cells have spread. Your doctor will probably do a complete physical examination as well, to judge your general health and to look for other evidence that the cancer may have spread.

If breast symptoms and/or the results of your physical examination suggest that breast cancer might be present, more tests will likely be done. These tests might include imaging tests, examining samples of nipple discharge, or biopsies of suspicious areas.

Imaging Tests Used to Evaluate Breast Disease

Imaging tests use x-rays, magnetic fields, sound waves, or radioactive substances to create pictures of the inside of your body. Imaging tests may be done to determine whether a suspicious area might be cancerous, to learn how far cancer has spread, or to help assess whether treatment is working.

Diagnostic mammograms

Although mammograms are mostly used for screening, they can also be used to examine the breast of a woman who has a breast problem. This problem can be a breast mass, nipple discharge, or an abnormality that was found on a screening mammogram. In some cases, special images known as **cone views with magnification** are used to make a small area of abnormal breast tissue easier to evaluate.

A diagnostic mammogram can show the following:

- The abnormality is not worrisome at all. In these cases, you can usually return to having routine yearly mammograms.
- The lesion (area of abnormal tissue) has a high likelihood of being benign (not cancerous). In these cases, you will probably return sooner than usual for your next mammogram, usually in 4 to 6 months.
- The lesion is more suspicious, and a biopsy is needed to determine whether it is cancerous.

Even if the mammogram shows no tumor, if you or your doctor can feel a lump, a biopsy will be needed to be certain it is not cancer. One exception would be if an ultrasound reveals that the lump is a simple cyst (a fluid-filled sac), which is very unlikely to be cancerous.

Digital mammograms: A **digital mammogram** (also known as a **full-field digital mammogram**, or **FFDM**) is like a standard mammogram in that x-rays are used to produce an image of the breast. The digital mammogram is different, however, in the way the image is recorded, viewed by the doctor, and stored. Standard mammograms are recorded on large sheets of photographic film. Digital mammograms are recorded and stored on a computer. After the examination, the doctor can view a digital mammogram on a computer screen and adjust the image size, brightness, or contrast to see specific areas more clearly. Digital images can also be sent electronically to another site for a remote consultation with breast specialists. Whereas many centers do not offer the digital option at this time, it is expected to become more widely available in the future.

Because digital mammograms cost more than standard mammograms, studies are now under way to determine which form of mammogram will ultimately be more beneficial to women. Some studies have found that women who have a digital mammogram are less likely to need additional imaging tests, owing to inconclusive results on the original mammogram. A recent large study found that a digital mammogram was more accurate in finding cancers in women younger than 50 and in women with dense breast tissue, although the rates of inconclusive results were similar between digital and standard mammography. It is important to remember that a standard mammogram also is effective for these groups of women and that they should not miss their regular mammogram if a digital mammogram is not available.

Computer-aided detection and diagnosis (CAD): Over the past 2 decades, computer-aided detection and diagnosis (CAD) has been developed to help radiologists detect suspicious changes on mammograms. This technique can be done with standard film mammograms or with digital mammograms.

Computers can help doctors identify abnormal areas on a mammogram by acting as a second set of eyes. For standard mammograms, the film is fed into a machine that converts the image into a digital signal. The digital signal is then analyzed by the computer. Alternatively, the technology can be applied to a digital mammogram. In that case, the computer displays the image on a video screen with markers pointing to areas that require closer examination by the radiologist.

The effectiveness of computer-aided detection and diagnosis remains unclear. Some doctors find it helpful, but a recent large study found it did not significantly improve the accuracy of breast cancer detection. It did, however, lead to an increase in the number of women needing breast biopsies. Further research is needed to determine the effectiveness of computer-aided tests for detecting breast cancer.

Magnetic resonance imaging of the breast

Magnetic resonance imaging (MRI) uses radio waves and strong magnets instead of x-rays. The energy from the radio waves is absorbed and then released in a pattern formed by the type of body tissue and by certain diseases. A computer translates the pattern into a very detailed image of parts of the body. A contrast liquid called gadolinium is often injected into a vein before or during the **scan** to show details more clearly.

An MRI can take a long time—often up to an hour. You have to lie inside a narrow tube, which is confining and may upset people with claustrophobia (a fear of enclosed spaces). The machine also makes loud buzzing and clicking noises that you may find disturbing. Some places will give you headphones with music to block this out. MRI scans are also expensive, although insurance plans generally pay for them when cancer has been diagnosed.

Although MRI machines are quite common, they need to be specifically adapted to look at the breast. Make sure that your medical facility is using one of these specially adapted machines.

MRI scans can be used in combination with mammograms for screening women who are at high risk for breast cancer, or it can be used to better examine suspicious areas found by a mammogram. Sometimes MRIs are used for guidance in biopsies of suspicious areas of the breast. This is discussed in more detail in the "Biopsy" section on pages 79–83. For women who have had breast cancer diagnosed, an MRI can help determine the actual size of the cancer and help find any other cancers in the breast.

Breast ultrasound

Ultrasound, also known as ultrasound scanning or ultrasonography, uses sound waves to outline a part of the body. For this test, a small, microphone-like instrument called a **transducer** is placed on the skin (after the skin is lubricated with ultrasound gel). The instrument emits sound waves and picks up the echoes as they bounce off body tissues. The echoes are converted by a computer into a black and white image that is displayed on a computer screen. This test is pain-less and does not expose you to radiation.

Ultrasound has become a valuable tool to use in combination with mammography because it is widely available and less expensive than other options, such as MRI. The use of ultrasound instead of mammograms for breast cancer **screening** is not recommended. Breast ultrasound is usually used to target a suspicious area found on the mammo-gram. Ultrasound helps distinguish between cysts (fluid-filled sacs) and solid masses and, sometimes, between benign and cancerous tumors.

Ultrasound may be most helpful in women with very dense breasts. Clinical trials are now looking at the benefits and risks of using breast ultrasound in combination with screening mammograms in women with dense breasts and a higher risk of breast cancer.

Ductogram

A **ductogram**, also called a **galactogram**, is sometimes helpful in determining the cause of nipple discharge. With this test, a very thin plastic tube is placed into the opening of the duct in the nipple. Local anesthesia may need to be used, depending on the difficulty of the tube insertion. A small amount of contrast medium is injected to outline the shape of the duct on an x-ray image and reveal whether there is a mass inside the duct.

Newer imaging tests

Newer tests such as **scintimammography** and **tomosynthesis** are not commonly used and are still being studied to determine their usefulness. They are described in more detail in the section, "What's New in Breast Cancer Research and Treatment?" on pages 231–243.

Other Tests

Some other tests may be done for the purposes of research, but they have not yet been found to be helpful in diagnosing breast cancer in most women.

Nipple discharge exam

If you are having nipple discharge, the doctor may collect some of the fluid and look at it under a microscope to see whether the fluid contains any cancer cells. Most nipple discharge or secretions are not cancerous. In general, if the secretion appears milky or clear green, cancer is very unlikely. If the discharge is red or reddish-brown, suggesting that it contains blood, it might be caused by cancer. However, an injury, infection, or benign tumor is more likely to be the cause.

Even when no cancer cells are found in the nipple discharge, it is not possible to say for certain that a breast cancer is not there. If a woman has a suspicious mass, it will be necessary to biopsy the mass, even if the nipple discharge does not contain cancer cells.

Ductal lavage and nipple aspiration

Ductal lavage is an experimental test developed for women who have no symptoms of breast cancer but are at very high risk for the disease. It is not a test to screen for or diagnose breast cancer, but it may help give a more accurate picture of a woman's cancer risk.

Ductal lavage can be done in a doctor's office or at an outpatient facility. An anesthetic cream is applied to numb the nipple area. Gentle suction is then used to help draw tiny amounts of fluid from the milk ducts up to the surface of the nipple, which helps the doctor locate the ducts' natural openings. A tiny tube (catheter) is then inserted into a duct opening. Saline (salt water solution) is slowly infused into the catheter to gently rinse the duct and collect cells. The ductal fluid is withdrawn through the catheter and sent to a laboratory, where the cells are examined under a microscope.

Ductal lavage is not appropriate for women who are not at high risk for breast cancer. The test has not been shown to be effective in detecting cancer early. It is more likely to be helpful as a test of breast cancer risk than as a screening test for cancer. More studies are needed to better define the usefulness of this test.

Nipple aspiration is also used to find abnormal cells developing in the ducts. However, this test is much simpler because nothing is inserted into the breast. The device for nipple aspiration uses small cups that are placed on the woman's breasts. The device warms the breasts, gently compresses them, and applies light suction to bring nipple fluid to the surface of the breast. The nipple fluid is then collected and sent to a laboratory for analysis. As with ductal lavage, the procedure may be useful as a test of cancer risk but is not appropriate as a screening test for cancer. The test has not been shown to detect cancer early.

Biopsy

During a **biopsy**, the doctor removes a sample from the suspicious area for examination under a microscope. A biopsy is done when mammograms, other imaging tests, or the physical examination finds a breast change or abnormality that could be cancer. A biopsy is the only way to determine whether cancer is really present.

There are several types of biopsies, such as **fine needle aspiration (FNA)** biopsy, core needle biopsy, and surgical biopsy. Each has advantages and disadvantages and should be discussed with your doctor. The choice of which to use depends on your specific situation. Your doctor will consider how suspicious the lesion appears, how large it is, its location in the breast, the number of lesions, other medical problems you may have, and your personal preferences.

Fine needle aspiration biopsy

With fine needle aspiration (FNA) biopsy, the doctor uses a very thin, hollow needle attached to a syringe to aspirate (withdraw) a small amount of tissue from a suspicious area. The tissue is then examined under a microscope. The needle used for FNA biopsies is thinner than a needle used for a blood test.

If the area to be biopsied can be felt, the doctor can guide the needle into the area while feeling it. If the lump cannot be easily felt, the doctor may use ultrasound to watch the needle on a screen as it moves toward and into the mass. A local **anesthetic** may be used. Because such a thin needle is used for the biopsy, the process of receiving the anesthetic may actually be more uncomfortable than the biopsy itself.

Once the needle is in place, fluid is withdrawn from the mass. If the fluid is clear, the lump is probably a benign cyst. Bloody or cloudy fluid can indicate a benign cyst or, very rarely, cancer. If the lump is solid, small tissue fragments are withdrawn. A pathologist will look at the biopsy tissue or fluid under a microscope to determine whether it is cancerous.

An FNA biopsy is the least complicated type of biopsy to have, but it has some disadvantages. Cancer can sometimes be missed if the needle is not placed among the cancer cells. And even if cancer cells are found, it is usually not possible to determine whether the cancer is invasive. In some cases, not enough cells are present to perform some of the other laboratory tests routinely done on breast cancer specimens. If the FNA biopsy does not provide a clear diagnosis or your doctor still has concerns, a second biopsy or a different type of biopsy should be done.

Core needle biopsy

With a **core needle biopsy**, a larger needle is used to take a tissue sample from an abnormal area felt by the doctor or pinpointed by ultrasound or mammogram. (When mammograms taken from different angles are used to pinpoint the biopsy site, this is known as a **stereotactic core needle biopsy**.) The biopsy is sometimes guided by an MRI scan.

The needle used in core biopsies is larger than that used in fine needle aspiration (FNA) biopsy. The needle removes a small cylinder, or core, of tissue (about $\frac{1}{16}$- to $\frac{1}{8}$-inch in diameter and $\frac{1}{2}$-inch long) from the suspicious area. Several tissue samples are usually removed. The biopsy is done by using local anesthesia (the patient is awake, but the breast is numbed) in an outpatient setting.

Because core needle biopsies remove larger pieces of tissue, they are more likely than FNA biopsies to provide a clear diagnosis. However, they may still miss some cancers.

Vacuum-assisted biopsies

Vacuum-assisted biopsies can be done with systems such as the Mammotome or ATEC (Automated Tissue Excision and Collection). For these procedures, the skin is numbed and a small incision (about $\frac{1}{4}$-inch long) is made. A hollow probe is inserted through the incision into the abnormal area of breast tissue. The probe can be guided into place by using x-rays, ultrasound, or, in the case of ATEC, an MRI. A cylinder of tissue is then suctioned in through a hole in the probe, and a rotating blade within the probe cuts the tissue sample from the rest of the breast. Several samples can be taken from the same incision. Vacuum-assisted biopsies are done as an outpatient procedure. No stitches are needed, and there is minimal scarring.

More tissue is usually removed with this method than with core needle biopsies.

Surgical biopsy

Sometimes surgery is needed to remove all or part of the lump for examination under a microscope. This is referred to as a **surgical biopsy** or an open biopsy. The surgical biopsy is usually an **excisional biopsy**, in which the surgeon removes the entire mass or abnormal area, as well as a surrounding margin of normal-appearing breast tissue. If the mass is too large to be removed easily, an **incisional biopsy** may be done instead. In an incisional biopsy, only part of the mass is removed. In rare cases, a surgical biopsy can be done in the doctor's office. More commonly, it is done in the hospital's outpatient department with the patient receiving local anesthesia. You may also be given medicine to make you drowsy. A surgical biopsy can also be done under general anesthesia (in which the patient is asleep).

During a surgical breast biopsy, the surgeon may use **stereotactic wire localization** if there is a small lump that is hard to locate by touch or if an area looks suspicious on the x-ray but a lump cannot be felt. With stereotactic wire localization, the area is numbed with local anesthesia and a thin hollow needle is placed into the breast. X-ray views are used to guide the needle to the suspicious area. Once the tip of the needle is in the right spot, a thin wire is inserted through the center of the needle. A small hook at the end of the wire keeps it in place while the hollow needle is removed. The surgeon can then use the wire as a guide to the abnormal area to be removed. The surgical specimen is sent to the laboratory to be examined under a microscope (see below, "Laboratory Examination of Breast Cancer Tissue").

A surgical biopsy is more complex than a fine needle aspiration biopsy or a core needle biopsy. It typically requires several stitches and may leave a scar. Core needle biopsy is usually enough to make a diagnosis, but sometimes a surgical biopsy may be needed if the core needle biopsy is inconclusive or the lesion is difficult to access by core needle biopsy.

Lymph node dissection and sentinel lymph node biopsy

Lymph node dissection and sentinel lymph node biopsy are done specifically to look for cancer in the lymph nodes. The section "How Is Breast Cancer Treated?" on pages 126–130 includes more detail about these procedures.

Laboratory Examination of Breast Cancer Tissue

Once samples of breast tissue have been obtained, they are examined in the laboratory to determine whether breast cancer is present and, if so, what type and grade of breast cancer it is. Other laboratory tests are performed to help determine how quickly a cancer is likely to grow and, to some extent, what treatments are likely to be effective.

If a benign condition is diagnosed, no further treatment is needed. Still, it is important to ask your doctor whether the benign condition places you at higher risk for breast cancer in the future and what type of follow-up care you might need.

If the diagnosis is cancer, you will have time to learn about the disease and to discuss treatment options with your **cancer care team**, friends, and family. It is usually not necessary to rush into treatment. You may want to get a second opinion before deciding what treatment is best for you.

Type of breast cancer

The breast tissue removed during the biopsy (or during surgery) is first examined under a microscope to determine whether cancer is present and whether it is noninvasive (in situ) or invasive. The biopsy is also used to determine the type of cancer. The most common types, invasive ductal carcinoma and invasive lobular carcinoma, generally are treated in the same way. The different types of breast cancer are defined in the section, "What Is Breast Cancer?" on pages 8–15.

Breast cancer grade

A pathologist also assigns a **grade** to the cancer, which is based on how closely the biopsy sample resembles normal breast tissue. The grade of cancer helps determine a woman's prognosis. In general, a lower grade indicates a slower-growing cancer that is less likely to spread, whereas a higher number indicates a faster-growing cancer that is more likely to spread. The tumor grade is one factor in determining the need for further treatment after surgery.

Histologic tumor grade (sometimes called the Bloom-Richardson grade, Scarff-Bloom-Richardson grade, or Elston-Ellis grade) is based on the frequency of cell division, or mitosis (the mitotic count); the percentage of the cancer that is composed of tubular structures; and how closely the cells resemble normal breast cells. This system of grading is used for invasive cancers but not for noninvasive (in situ) cancers.

- **Grade 1** (well-differentiated) cancers have relatively normal-looking cells that do not appear to be growing rapidly and are arranged in small tubules.
- **Grade 2** (moderately differentiated) cancers have features between grades 1 and 3.
- **Grade 3** (poorly differentiated) cancers, the highest grade, lack normal features and tend to grow and spread more aggressively.

Ductal carcinoma in situ (DCIS) is sometimes assigned a **nuclear grade**, which describes how abnormal the cancer cells appear. The presence or absence of necrosis (areas of dead or degenerating cancer cells), which might indicate a more aggressive cancer, is also noted. Other factors important in determining the prognosis for DCIS include the **surgical margin** (how close the cancer is to the edge of the specimen) and the size (amount of breast tissue affected by DCIS). In situ cancers with a high nuclear grade, necrosis, cancer at or near the edge of the sample, or large areas (more involvement) of DCIS are more likely to recur after treatment.

Estrogen receptor and progesterone receptor status

Receptors are proteins on the outside surfaces of cells that can attach to certain substances, such as hormones, that circulate in the blood. Normal breast cells and some breast cancer cells have receptors that attach to estrogen and progesterone—the 2 hormones that often fuel the growth of breast cancer cells.

An important step in evaluating a breast cancer is to test a portion of the cancer removed during the biopsy or surgery for the presence of estrogen and progesterone receptors. Cancer cells may contain neither, one, or both of these receptors. Breast cancers that contain estrogen receptors are often referred to as "ER–positive" (or ER+) cancers, whereas those containing progesterone receptors are called "PR–positive" (or PR+) cancers. Women with hormone receptor–positive cancers tend to have a better prognosis and are much more likely to respond to hormone therapy than women with cancers without these receptors.

All breast cancers, with the exception of lobular carcinoma in situ (LCIS), should be tested for these hormone receptors at the time of the breast biopsy or surgery. Approximately 2 of 3 breast cancers contain at least one of these receptors. This percentage is higher in older women than in younger women.

HER2/neu status

About 1 of every 5 breast cancers has too much of a growth-promoting protein called HER2/neu (often just shortened to HER2). This protein is made by cells under the instruction of the HER2/neu gene. Tumors with increased levels of HER2/neu are referred to as "HER2-positive."

Women with HER2-positive breast cancer have too many copies of the HER2/neu gene, resulting in greater than normal amounts of the HER2/neu protein. These cancers tend to grow and spread more aggressively than other types of breast cancer.

All newly diagnosed breast cancers should be tested for HER2/neu because HER2-positive cancers are much more likely to benefit from treatment with drugs that target the HER2/neu protein, such as trastuzumab (Herceptin) and lapatinib (Tykerb). For more information on these drugs, see the section "How Is Breast Cancer Treated?" on pages 157–159.

Testing of the biopsy or surgery sample is usually done in one of two ways:

- **immunohistochemistry (IHC):** In this test, special antibodies that identify the HER2/neu protein are applied to the sample, and these antibodies cause cells to change color if many copies are present. This color change can be seen under a microscope. The test results are reported as 0, 1+, 2+, or 3+.
- **fluorescence in situ hybridization (FISH):** This test uses fluorescent pieces of DNA that specifically stick to copies of the HER2/neu gene in cells, which can then be counted under a special microscope.

Many breast cancer specialists agree that the FISH test is more accurate than IHC. However, it is more expensive, and it takes longer to get the results. The IHC test is often used first. If the results are 0 or 1+, the cancer is considered HER2-negative. People with HER2-negative tumors are not treated with drugs that target HER2 (such as trastuzumab). If the result is 2+, the HER2 status of the tumor is not clear. In this case, the tumor may be tested with FISH. If the test result is 3+, the cancer is considered HER2-positive. Patients with HER2-positive tumors may be treated with drugs such as trastuzumab. Newer test methods are now becoming available as well (see the section "What's New in Breast Cancer Research and Treatment?" on pages 231–243).

Tests of ploidy and cell proliferation rate

The **ploidy** of cancer cells refers to the amount of DNA they contain. If there is a normal amount of DNA in the cells, they are said to be **diploid**. If the amount is abnormal, then the cells are described as **aneuploid**. Although tests of ploidy may help determine prognosis, they rarely change treatment and are considered optional. They are not usually recommended as part of a routine breast cancer work-up.

The **S-phase fraction** is the percentage of cells in a sample that are replicating (copying) their DNA. DNA replication occurs when the cell divides into 2 new cells. The rate of cancer cell division can also be estimated by a **Ki-67** test. A high S-phase fraction or high Ki-67 labeling index means that the cancer cells are dividing more rapidly, which indicates a more aggressive cancer.

Tests of gene patterns

Researchers have found that looking at the patterns of a number of different genes at the same time (sometimes referred to as gene expression profiling) can help predict whether an early-stage breast cancer is likely to recur after initial treatment. Two such tests, which look at different sets of genes, are now available.

Oncotype DX: The Oncotype DX test may be helpful when deciding whether additional treatment with chemotherapy after surgery (called adjuvant chemotherapy) might be useful in women with certain early-stage breast cancers that usually have a low chance of recurrence (such as stage I or II estrogen receptor–positive breast cancers without lymph node involvement). Recent studies have shown that this test may also be helpful for patients with lymph node involvement.

The Oncotype DX test looks at a set of 21 genes in cells from tumor samples to determine a recurrence score—a number between 0 and 100:

- Women with a score of 17 or below have a low risk of recurrence.
- Women with a score of 18 to 30 are at intermediate risk.
- Women with a score of 31 or more are at high risk.

The test cannot reveal with certainty whether cancer will recur in an individual. The test is a tool that can be used, along with other factors, to help guide women and their doctors when deciding whether more treatment might be useful.

MammaPrint: The **MammaPrint** test can be used to help determine the likelihood that certain early-stage breast cancers (stage I or II) will recur in a distant part of the body after treatment. It can be used for either ER–negative or ER–positive tumors. The test is used to examine the activity of 70 different genes to determine whether the risk of recurrence is low or high. This information can help doctors decide whether adjuvant (additional) treatment is needed. With a MammaPrint test, the tumor must be collected and stored in a certain way, so the decision to do this test must be made before surgery.

Usefulness of these tests: Whereas some doctors are using the Oncotype DX and MammaPrint tests (along with other resources) as they make decisions about offering chemotherapy, others are waiting for more research to prove they are helpful. Large clinical trials of these tests are now being done. In the meantime, women should ask their doctors whether these tests could be useful for them.

How Is Breast Cancer Staged?

The **stage** describes the extent of the cancer in the body. It is based on whether the cancer is invasive or noninvasive, the size of the tumor, how many lymph nodes are involved, and whether it has spread to other parts of the body. The stage of a cancer is one of the most important factors in determining prognosis and treatment options.

Staging is the process of finding out how widespread a cancer is when it is diagnosed. Depending on the results of your physical examination and biopsy, your doctor may want you to have certain imaging tests such as a chest x-ray, mammograms of both breasts, bone scans, computed tomography (CT) scans, magnetic resonance imaging (MRI), and/or positron emission tomography (PET) scans (described in detail in the next section). Blood tests may also be done to evaluate your overall health and help find out whether the cancer has spread to certain organs.

Imaging Tests for Detecting Metastasis in Breast Cancer

Once breast cancer is diagnosed, one or more of the following tests may be done to detect cancer cells that may have metastasized (spread) to other places in the body.

Chest x-ray

A chest x-ray may be done to see whether the breast cancer has spread to your lungs.

Mammogram

Extensive mammograms may be done to obtain thorough views of the breasts and check for any other abnormal areas that could be cancerous. The section "How Is Breast Cancer Diagnosed?" includes more information about this test.

Bone scan

A **bone scan** can help reveal whether cancer has spread to your bones. Bone scans can be more useful than standard x-rays because they can show all of the bones of the body at the same time. For this test, a small amount of low-level radioactive material is injected into a vein (by an **intravenous**, or **IV**, **line**). Over the course of a couple of hours, the substance settles in areas of bone change throughout the skeleton. You then lie on a table for about 30 minutes while a special camera detects the radioactivity and creates a picture of your skeleton. Areas of bone change (which attract the radioactive material) appear as "**hot spots**" on your skeleton. These areas may suggest the presence of metastatic cancer, but arthritis or other bone diseases can also cause the same pattern. To distinguish between these conditions, your cancer care team may use other imaging tests or they may take a bone biopsy.

Computed tomography

A **computed tomography (CT) scan** is an x-ray procedure that produces detailed cross-sectional images of the body. Instead of taking one picture, like a regular x-ray, a CT scanner takes many pictures as it rotates around you while you lie on a table. A computer then combines these pictures into images of slices of the part of your body being studied. In women with breast cancer, this test is most often used to look at the chest and/or abdomen to see if the cancer has spread to other organs.

Before the CT scan, you may be asked to drink 1 to 2 pints of a contrast solution. The contrast solution helps outline the intestines so that certain areas are not mistaken for tumors. You may also receive an IV line through which a different kind of contrast dye (IV contrast) is injected. The contrast dye helps outline structures in your body.

The contrast solution may cause some flushing (a feeling of warmth, especially in the face). Some people are allergic to the solution and get hives. Rarely, more serious reactions such as trouble breathing or low blood pressure can occur. Medicine can prevent and treat allergic reactions. Be sure to tell the doctor if you have ever had a reaction to any contrast material used for x-rays.

CT scans take longer than regular x-rays. You will lie still on a table for 15 to 30 minutes while the scans are being done. During the test, the table moves in and out of the scanner, a ring-shaped machine that completely surrounds the table. You may feel confined by the equipment while the pictures are being taken.

CT-guided needle biopsy: CT scans can also be used to precisely guide a biopsy needle into a suspected area of cancer metastasis. For this procedure, you remain on the CT scanning table while a radiologist advances a biopsy needle through the skin and toward the location of the mass. CT scans are repeated until the doctors are sure that the needle is within the mass. A fine needle biopsy sample (a tiny fragment of tissue) or a core needle biopsy sample (a thin cylinder of tissue about ½-inch long and less than ⅛-inch in diameter) is then removed and sent to the laboratory for examination.

Magnetic resonance imaging

Magnetic resonance imaging (MRI) is described as an imaging test in the sections "Can Breast Cancer Be Found Early?" (pages 44–68) and "How Is Breast Cancer Diagnosed?" (pages 69–90). An MRI may be used to examine the breast with cancer to look for other tumors. It may also be used to look at the opposite breast to determine whether it contains any tumors. It is not clear how helpful MRI is in planning surgery in someone known to have breast cancer. Like CT scans, MRI is also used to determine whether cancer has spread to various parts of the body. MRI scans are particularly helpful in looking at the brain and spinal cord.

MRI scans use radio waves and very strong magnets instead of x-rays. The energy from the radio waves is absorbed and then released in a pattern formed by the type of body tissue and by certain diseases. A computer translates the pattern into a very detailed image of parts of the body. A contrast material called gadolinium is often injected into a vein before the scan to better view the details.

MRI scans are a little more uncomfortable than CT scans. First, they take longer—often up to an hour. Second, you have to lie inside a narrow tube, which is confining and can upset people with claustrophobia (a fear of enclosed spaces). Newer, "open" MRI machines can alleviate this problem. The machine also makes buzzing and clicking noises that might be disturbing to some people. Some centers provide headphones with music to block out these sounds.

Ultrasound

In the section "How Is Breast Cancer Diagnosed?"(pages 75–76), ultrasound is described as an imaging test of the breast. However, ultrasound can also be used to determine whether cancer has spread to other parts of the body.

Ultrasound tests use sound waves and their echoes to produce a picture of internal organs or masses. A small microphone-like instrument called a **transducer** sends out sound waves and picks up the echoes as they bounce off body tissues. The echoes are converted by a computer into a black and white image that is shown on a computer screen. This test is painless and does not expose you to radiation. Abdominal ultrasound can be used to look for tumors in the liver or other abdominal organs. In an abdominal ultrasound, the person lies on a table. The skin is usually lubricated with gel. A technician then moves a transducer over the skin overlying the part of the body being examined.

Positron emission tomography

For a **positron emission tomography (PET)** scan, glucose (a form of sugar) that contains a radioactive atom is injected into the bloodstream. Cancer cells in the body absorb large amounts of the radioactive sugar. After about an hour, a special camera is used to create a picture of areas of radioactivity in the body.

A PET scan can be useful when your doctor believes the cancer may have spread but the location is unknown. The picture is not finely detailed like a CT or MRI scan, but it provides helpful information about your whole body. Some newer machines are able to do both a PET and CT scan at the same time. This combination allows the radiologist to compare areas of higher radioactivity on the PET scan with the appearance of that area on the CT scan. So far, most studies show that a PET scan is not very helpful in most cases of breast cancer, although it may be used when the cancer is known to have spread.

The American Joint Committee on Cancer TNM System

A staging system is a standardized way for the cancer care team to summarize information about how far a cancer has spread.

The most common system used to describe the stages of breast cancer is the **American Joint Committee on Cancer (AJCC) TNM system**. The stage of a breast cancer can be based either on the results of physical examination, biopsy, and imaging tests (called the **clinical stage**), or on the results of these tests plus the results of surgery (called the **pathologic stage**). The staging described here is the pathologic stage, which includes the findings after surgery, when the pathologist has examined the breast mass and nearby lymph nodes. Pathologic staging is likely to be more accurate than clinical staging because it allows the doctor to get a firsthand impression of the extent of the cancer.

The TNM staging system classifies cancers based on their T, N, and M stages:

- The letter **T** followed by a number from 0 to 4 describes the tumor's size and spread to the skin or to the chest wall under the breast. Higher T numbers mean a larger tumor and/or wider spread to tissues near the breast.
- The letter **N** followed by a number from 0 to 3 indicates whether the cancer has spread to lymph nodes near the breast and, if so, how many lymph nodes are affected.
- The letter **M** followed by a 0 or 1 indicates whether the cancer has spread to distant organs, such as the lungs or bones.

Primary tumor (T) categories:

TX: Primary tumor cannot be assessed.

T0: No evidence of primary tumor found.

Tis: Carcinoma in situ (DCIS, LCIS, or Paget disease of the nipple with no associated tumor mass) is present.

T1: Tumor is 2 cm (¾ of an inch) or less across.

T2: Tumor is more than 2 cm but not more than 5 cm (2 inches) across.

T3: Tumor is more than 5 cm across.

T4: Tumor of any size is growing into the chest wall or skin. This includes inflammatory breast cancer.

Nearby lymph nodes (N) (based on examination under a microscope): Lymph node staging for breast cancer has changed over time as technology has evolved. Earlier methods were useful in finding large deposits of cancer cells in the lymph nodes but could miss microscopic areas of cancer spread. Over time, newer methods have made it possible to find much smaller deposits of cancer cells. However, experts have not been sure of how to interpret this new information. Do tiny deposits of cancer cells affect prognosis in the same way that larger deposits do? How much cancer in the lymph node is needed to change prognosis or treatment?

While these questions are still under study, the current consensus is that an area of cancer cells must contain at least 200 cells or be at least 0.2 mm across (less than $\frac{1}{100}$ of an inch) for the N stage to change. An area of cancer metastasis smaller than 0.2 mm (or having fewer than 200 cells) does not change the stage. However, an abbreviation is added to the stage that reflects the way the metastasis was detected. The abbreviation "i+" means that cancer cells were only seen when a special technique, called immunohistochemistry, was used. The abbreviation "mol+" is used if the cancer cells were only seen using a technique called PCR. These very tiny areas are sometimes called isolated tumor cells.

If the area of cancer spread is between 0.2 mm (or 200 cells) and 2 mm (about the width of 2 grains of rice), it is called a micrometastasis. Micrometastases change the N stage. Areas of metastasis larger than 2 mm affect prognosis and also change the N stage. A larger area is sometimes called a macrometastasis but may just be called a metastasis.

NX: Nearby lymph nodes cannot be assessed (for example, removed previously).

N0: Cancer has not spread to nearby lymph nodes.

> **N0(i+)**: Tiny amounts of cancer are found in axillary (underarm) lymph nodes by using immunohistochemistry. The area of metastasis contains fewer than 200 cells and is smaller than 0.2 mm.

> **N0(mol+)**: Cancer cells cannot be seen in axillary lymph nodes using immunohistochemistry, but traces of cancer cells were detected using the PCR test.

N1: Cancer has spread to 1 to 3 axillary (underarm) lymph node(s), and/or tiny amounts of cancer are found in internal mammary lymph nodes (those near the breastbone) on sentinel lymph node biopsy.

> **N1mi**: Micrometastases (tiny areas of cancer spread) are found in 1 to 3 axillary lymph nodes. The areas of metastasis in the lymph nodes are 2 mm or smaller in size (but contain at least 200 cancer cells or are at least 0.2 mm in size).

N1a: Cancer has spread to 1 to 3 axillary lymph nodes with at least one area of metastasis larger than 2 mm.

N1b: Cancer has spread to internal mammary lymph nodes, but this spread could only be detected through sentinel lymph node biopsy and did not cause the lymph nodes to become enlarged.

N1c: Both N1a and N1b apply.

N2: Cancer has spread to 4 to 9 axillary lymph nodes or cancer has enlarged the internal mammary lymph nodes (either N2a or N2b, but not both).

N2a: Cancer has spread to 4 to 9 axillary lymph nodes, with at least one area of metastasis larger than 2 mm.

N2b: Cancer has spread to one or more internal mammary lymph nodes, causing them to become enlarged.

N3: Any of the following statements applies:

N3a: Either—

- Cancer has spread to 10 or more axillary lymph nodes, with at least one area of metastasis larger than 2 mm.

OR

- Cancer has spread to the lymph nodes under the clavicle (collarbone), with at least one area of metastasis larger than 2 mm.

N3b: Either—

- Cancer is found in at least one axillary lymph node (with at least one area of metastasis larger than 2 mm) and has enlarged the internal mammary lymph nodes.

OR

- Cancer involves 4 or more axillary lymph nodes (with at least one area of metastasis larger than 2 mm), and tiny amounts of cancer are found in internal mammary lymph nodes on sentinel lymph node biopsy.

N3c: Cancer has spread to the lymph nodes above the clavicle with at least one area of metastasis larger than 2 mm.

Metastasis (M):

MX: Presence of distant metastasis cannot be assessed.

M0: No distant metastasis is found on x-rays or other imaging procedures or by physical exam.

cM0(i +): Small numbers of cancer cells are found in blood or bone marrow or tiny areas of metastasis (0.2 mm or smaller) are found in any lymph nodes.

M1: Spread to distant organs is present. (The most common sites are bone, lung, brain, and liver.)

Breast Cancer Stage Grouping

Once the T, N, and M categories have been determined, this information is combined in a process called stage grouping. Cancers with similar stages tend to have a similar prognosis and thus are often treated in a similar way. Stage is expressed in Roman numerals from stage I (the least advanced stage) to stage IV (the most advanced stage). Noninvasive cancer is listed as stage 0.

Stage 0: Tis, N0, M0

Stage 0 refers to ductal carcinoma in situ (DCIS), the earliest form of breast cancer. In DCIS, cancer cells are still within a duct and have not invaded the surrounding fatty breast tissue. Lobular carcinoma in situ (LCIS) is sometimes also classified as stage 0 breast cancer, but most oncologists believe it is not a true breast cancer. In LCIS, abnormal cells grow within the lobules, but they do not penetrate through the walls of the lobules. Paget disease of the nipple (without an underlying tumor mass) is also stage 0. In all these cases, the cancer has not spread to lymph nodes or distant sites.

Stage IA: T1, N0, M0

The tumor is 2 cm (about ¾ of an inch) or less across (T1) and has not spread to lymph nodes (N0) or distant sites (M0).

Stage IB: T0 or T1, N1mi, M0

The tumor is 2 cm or less across (or is not found) (T0 or T1) with micrometastases in 1 to 3 axillary lymph nodes (the cancer in the lymph nodes is greater than 0.2 mm across and/or more than 200 cells but is not larger than 2 mm) (N1mi).

The cancer has not spread to distant sites (M0).

Stage IIA: One of the following applies:

T0 or T1, N1 (but not N1mi), M0: The tumor is 2 cm or less across (or is not found) (T1 or T0) and either:

- It has spread to 1 to 3 axillary lymph nodes, with the cancer in the lymph nodes larger than 2 mm across (N1a).

OR

- Tiny amounts of cancer are found in internal mammary lymph nodes on sentinel lymph node biopsy (N1b).

OR

- It has spread to 1 to 3 lymph nodes under the arm and to internal mammary lymph nodes (found on sentinel lymph node biopsy) (N1c).

OR

T2, N0, M0: The tumor is larger than 2 cm across and less than 5 cm (T2) but hasn't spread to the lymph nodes (N0).

The cancer has not spread to distant sites (M0).

Stage IIB: One of the following applies:

T2, N1, M0: The tumor is larger than 2 cm and less than 5 cm across (T2). It has spread to 1 to 3 axillary lymph nodes and/or tiny amounts of cancer are found in internal mammary lymph nodes on sentinel lymph node biopsy (N1).

The cancer has not spread to distant sites (M0).

OR

T3, N0, M0: The tumor is larger than 5 cm across but does not grow into the chest wall or skin and has not spread to lymph nodes (T3, N0).

The cancer has not spread to distant sites (M0).

Stage IIIA: One of the following applies:

T0 to T2, N2, M0: The tumor is not more than 5 cm across (or cannot be found) (T0 to T2). It has spread to 4 to 9 axillary lymph nodes, or it has enlarged the internal mammary lymph nodes (N2).

The cancer has not spread to distant sites (M0).

OR

T3, N1 or N2, M0: The tumor is larger than 5 cm across but does not grow into the chest wall or skin (T3). It has spread to 1 to 9 axillary nodes, or to internal mammary nodes (N1 or N2).

The cancer has not spread to distant sites (M0).

Stage IIIB: T4, N0 to N2, M0

The tumor has grown into the chest wall or skin (T4), and one of the following statements applies:

- It has not spread to lymph nodes (N0).
- It has spread to 1 to 3 axillary lymph nodes and/or tiny amounts of cancer are found in internal mammary lymph nodes on sentinel lymph node biopsy (N1).
- It has spread to 4 to 9 axillary lymph nodes, or it has enlarged the internal mammary lymph nodes (N2).

The cancer has not spread to distant sites (M0).

Inflammatory breast cancer is classified as T4 and is stage IIIB unless it has spread to distant lymph nodes or organs, in which case it would be stage IV.

Stage IIIC: any T, N3, M0

The tumor is any size (or cannot be found), and one of the following statements applies:

- Cancer has spread to 10 or more axillary lymph nodes (N3).
- Cancer has spread to the lymph nodes under the clavicle (N3).
- Cancer has spread to the lymph nodes above the clavicle (N3).
- Cancer involves axillary lymph nodes and has enlarged the internal mammary lymph nodes (N3).
- Cancer has spread to 4 or more axillary lymph nodes, and tiny amounts of cancer are found in internal mammary lymph nodes on sentinel lymph node biopsy (N3).

The cancer has not spread to distant sites (M0).

Stage IV: any T, any N, M1

The cancer can be any size (any T) and may or may not have spread to nearby lymph nodes (any N). It has spread to distant organs or to lymph nodes far from the breast (M1). The most common sites of metastasis are the bones, liver, brain, and lung.

If you have any questions about the stage of your cancer and what it might mean in your case, ask your doctor.

Breast Cancer Survival Rates by Stage

The numbers included in the table on page 107 come from the National Cancer Data Base and are based on people whose breast cancer was diagnosed in 2001 and 2002. Here are some important points to understand about these numbers:

- The **5-year survival rate** refers to the percentage of patients who live at least 5 years after receiving a diagnosis of breast cancer. Many of these patients live much longer than 5 years after diagnosis. Also, people who have a breast cancer diagnosis can die of other causes, and these numbers do not account for this fact.

- This database does not divide survival rates by all of the substages, such as IA and IB. The rates for these substages are likely to be close to the rate for the overall stage. For example, the survival rate for stage IA is likely to be slightly higher than that listed for stage I, whereas the survival rate for stage IB would be expected to be slightly lower.

- These numbers were taken from patients treated several years ago. Although they are among the most current numbers available, improvements in treatment since then mean that the survival rates for people receiving cancer diagnoses now may be higher.

- Whereas survival statistics can sometimes be useful as a general guide, they may not accurately represent any one person's prognosis. A number of other factors, including other tumor characteristics and a person's age and general health, can also affect prognosis. Your doctor can tell you how these numbers may apply to you, as he or she is familiar with the aspects of your particular situation.

Stage	5-year Survival Rate
0	93%
I	88%
IIA	81%
IIB	74%
IIIA	67%
IIIB	41%*
IIIC	49%*
IV	15%

*These numbers are correct as written (stage IIIB shows worse survival than stage IIIC).

Treatment

How Is Breast Cancer Treated?

This section begins with an overview of members of your cancer care team. You may see a number of doctors and health care professionals over the course of your diagnosis and treatment, and this section summarizes some of the key professionals who may be part of your care. The different types of treatment used for breast cancer and the typical treatment options based on the stage of the cancer are discussed beginning on page 117. These are followed by a small section on breast cancer during pregnancy and a section on breast reconstruction.

Your Cancer Care Team

Your cancer care team comprises several people, each with a different type of expertise to contribute to your care. One of your team members will take the lead in coordinating your care. Most breast cancer patients choose a medical oncologist or breast specialist to lead the team. It should be clear to all team members who is in charge, and that person should inform the others of your progress.

This alphabetical list will acquaint you with the health care professionals you may encounter, depending on which treatment option and

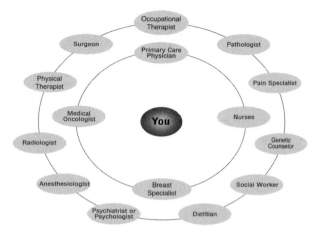

follow-up path you choose, and their areas of expertise.

Anesthesiologist

An anesthesiologist is a medical doctor who administers **anesthesia** (drugs or gases) to make you sleep and be unconscious or to prevent or relieve pain during and after a surgical procedure.

Breast specialist

A breast specialist is a doctor who specializes in the diagnosis and treatment of disorders of the breast.

Dietitian

A dietitian is specially trained to help you make healthy diet choices and maintain a healthy weight before, during, and after treatment. Dietitians can help patients deal with side effects of treatment, such as nausea, vomiting, or sore throat. A registered dietitian (RD) has at least a bachelor's degree and has passed a national competency exam.

Genetic counselor

A genetic counselor is a health care professional trained to help people through the process of genetic testing. A genetic counselor can explain the available tests to you, discuss the pros and cons, and address any concerns you might have. This counselor can arrange for genetic testing and then help interpret the test results. A certified genetic counselor has at least a master's degree and has passed both a general competency examination and a specialty **genetic counseling** examination.

Medical oncologist

A medical oncologist (also sometimes called an oncologist) is a medical doctor you may see after diagnosis. The oncologist is a cancer expert who understands specific types of cancer, their treatments, and their causes. He or she may help cancer patients make decisions about a course of treatment and then manage all phases of cancer care. Oncologists most often become involved when you need chemotherapy, but can also prescribe hormone therapy and other anticancer drugs.

Nurses

During your treatment you will be in contact with different types of nurses.

Case manager: The case manager is usually a nurse or oncology nurse specialist, who coordinates the patient's care throughout diagnosis, treatment, and recovery. The case manager provides guidance through the complex health care system by cutting through red tape, getting responses to questions, managing crises, and connecting the patient and family to needed resources.

Clinical nurse specialist: A clinical nurse specialist (CNS) is a nurse who has a master's degree in a specific area, such as oncology, psychiatry, or critical care nursing. The CNS often provides expertise to staff and may provide special services to patients, such as leading support groups and coordinating cancer care.

Nurse practitioner: A nurse practitioner is a registered nurse with a master's degree or doctoral degree who can manage the care of patients with breast cancer and has additional training in primary care. He or she shares many tasks with your doctors, such as recording your medical history, conducting physical examinations, and doing follow-up care. In most states, a nurse practitioner can prescribe medications with a doctor's supervision.

Oncology-certified nurse: An oncology-certified nurse is a registered nurse who has demonstrated an in-depth knowledge of oncology care. He or she has passed a certification examination. Oncology-certified nurses are found in all areas of cancer practice.

Registered nurse: A registered nurse has an associate or bachelor's degree in nursing and has passed a state licensing exam. He or she can monitor your condition, provide treatment, educate you about side effects, and help you adjust to cancer, both physically and emotionally.

Occupational therapist

An occupational therapist is a health care professional who helps restore self care, work, or leisure skills. They generally have a 4-year degree and are certified.

Pain specialist

Pain specialists are doctors, nurses, and pharmacists who are experts in managing pain. They can help you find pain control methods that are effective and allow you to maintain your **quality of life**. Not all doctors and nurses are trained in pain care, so you may have to request a pain specialist if your pain relief needs are not being met.

Pathologist

A pathologist is a medical doctor specially trained in diagnosing disease based on examination of microscopic tissue and fluid samples. He or she will determine the classification (cell type) of your cancer, help determine the stage (extent) and grade (estimate of aggressiveness) of your cancer, and issue a pathology report so that you and your doctor can decide on treatment options.

Personal or primary care physician

A personal physician may be a general doctor, internist, or family practice doctor. He or she is often the medical doctor you first saw when you noticed symptoms of illness. This general or family practice doctor may be a member of your medical team, but a specialist is most often a patient's cancer care team leader.

Physician assistant: Physician assistants (PAs) are health care professionals licensed to practice medicine with physician supervision. Physician assistants practice in the areas of primary care medicine (family medicine, internal medicine, pediatrics, and obstetrics and gynecology), as well as in surgery and the surgical subspecialties. Under the supervision of a doctor, they can diagnose and treat medical problems and, in most states, can also prescribe medications.

Physical therapist

A physical therapist is a health care professional who helps restore, maintain, and promote overall fitness and health.

Psychologist or psychiatrist

A psychologist is a licensed mental health professional who is often part of the cancer care team. He or she provides counseling on emotional and psychological issues. A psychologist may have specialized training and experience in treating people with cancer. A psychiatrist is a medical doctor specializing in mental health and behavioral disorders. Psychiatrists provide counseling and can also prescribe medications.

Radiologist

A radiologist is a medical doctor specializing in the use of imaging procedures (for example, diagnostic x-rays, ultrasound, magnetic resonance images, and bone scans) that produce pictures of internal body structures. He or she has special training in diagnosing cancer and other diseases and interpreting the results of imaging procedures. Your radiologist issues a radiology report describing the findings to your breast specialist or radiation oncologist. The radiology images and report may be used to aid in diagnosis; to help classify and determine the extent of your illness; to help locate tumors during procedures, surgery, and radiation treatment; or to look for the possible spread or recurrence of the cancer after treatment.

Radiation oncologist: A radiation oncologist is a medical doctor who specializes in treating cancer by using therapeutic radiation (high-energy x-rays or seeds). If you choose radiation, the radiation oncologist evaluates you frequently during the course of treatment and at intervals afterward. The radiation oncologist will usually work closely with your oncologist and will help you make decisions about radiation therapy options. A radiation oncologist is assisted by a radiation therapist during treatment and works with a radiation physicist, an expert who is trained in ensuring that you receive the correct dose of radiation treatment. The physicist is also assisted by a dosimetrist, a technician who helps plan and calculate the dosage, number, and length of your radiation treatments.

Radiation physicist: A radiation physicist ensures that the radiation machine delivers the right amount of radiation to the correct site in the body. The physicist works with the radiation oncologist to choose the treatment schedule and dose that will have the best chance of killing the most cancer cells.

Social worker

A social worker is a health specialist, usually with a master's degree, who is licensed or certified by the state in which he or she works. A social worker is an expert in coordinating and providing social services. He or she is trained to help you and your family deal with a range of emotional and practical challenges, such as finances, child care, emotional issues, family concerns and relationships, transportation, and problems with the health care system. If your social worker is trained in cancer-related problems, he or she can counsel you about your fears or concerns, help answer questions about diagnosis and treatment, and lead cancer support groups. You may communicate with your social worker during a hospital stay or on an outpatient basis.

Surgeon

Several different types of surgeons provide treatment for breast cancer. A general surgeon is trained to operate on all parts of the body. A surgical oncologist is a surgeon who has had advanced training in the surgical treatment of people with cancer. Cancer centers usually have one or more such individuals on their staff. A breast surgeon is a surgeon who has had advanced training in the surgical treatment of people with breast disorders or diseases.

Although each type of surgeon has a different area of expertise, each plays the same role in treating people with breast cancer. If you require surgery as part of your treatment, the surgeon will perform the operation and then manage any side effects you might have. He or she will also issue a report to your other doctors to help determine the rest of your treatment plan.

General Types of Treatment

Treatments can be classified into broad groups, based on how they work and when they are used.

Local versus systemic therapy

Local therapy is intended to treat a tumor at the site without affecting the rest of the body. Surgery and radiation therapy are examples of local therapies.

Systemic therapy refers to drugs that can be given by mouth or directly into the bloodstream to reach cancer cells anywhere in the body. Chemotherapy, hormone therapy, and **targeted therapy** are systemic therapies.

Adjuvant and neoadjuvant therapy

Women who have no detectable cancer after surgery are often given **adjuvant** (additional) **therapy**. In some cases, cancer cells break away from the primary breast tumor and begin to spread through the body by way of the bloodstream, even in the early stages of the disease. These cells cause no symptoms and cannot be felt on a physical examination or seen on x-rays or other imaging tests. However, they can establish new tumors in other organs or in bones. The goal of adjuvant therapy is to kill these hidden cells.

Not every person needs adjuvant therapy. Generally speaking, if the tumor is large or the cancer has spread to lymph nodes, it is more likely to have spread through the bloodstream. There are other features, some of which have already been discussed, that may determine whether the person should get adjuvant therapy. Recommendations about adjuvant therapy are discussed in the sections on specific treatments and in the section on treatment by stage.

Some women are given treatment such as chemotherapy or hormone therapy before surgery to shrink a tumor in the hope that a less extensive operation will be needed. This approach is called **neoadjuvant therapy**.

Surgery for Breast Cancer

Most women with breast cancer have some type of surgery. Surgery is often needed to remove a breast tumor, either breast-conserving surgery or mastectomy. Breast reconstruction can be done at the same time as the mastectomy or later. Surgery is also used to check the axillary lymph nodes for metastasis, either by sentinel lymph node biopsy or axillary lymph node dissection.

Breast-conserving surgery

In breast-conserving surgery, which is sometimes called **partial** or **segmental mastectomy**, only part of the affected breast is removed. The size and location of the tumor (and other factors) will dictate how much of the breast is removed. If radiation therapy is to be given after breast-conserving surgery, small metallic clips (which will be visible on x-rays) may be placed inside the breast during surgery to mark the area for the radiation treatments.

A **lumpectomy** removes only the breast lump and a surrounding margin of normal tissue. Radiation therapy is usually given after a lumpectomy. If adjuvant chemotherapy is to be given as well, radiation is usually delayed until the chemotherapy is completed.

A partial (segmental) mastectomy or **quadrantectomy** removes more breast tissue than a lumpectomy. With a quadrantectomy, one quarter of the breast is removed. Radiation therapy is usually given after surgery. Again, radiation may be delayed if chemotherapy is to be given as well.

If the pathologist finds cancer cells at the margin (the edge) of the piece of tissue removed, it is said to have positive margins. If no cancer cells are found at the edges of the tissue, it is said to have negative or clear margins. A positive margin means that some cancer cells may have been left behind after surgery, and the surgeon may need to go back and remove more tissue. This operation is called a **reexcision**. If the surgeon cannot remove enough breast tissue to get clear surgical margins, a mastectomy may be needed.

For most women with stage I or II breast cancer, breast-conservation therapy (lumpectomy or partial mastectomy plus radiation therapy) is as effective as mastectomy. Survival rates are the same for women treated with these 2 approaches. However, breast-conservation therapy is not an option for all women with breast cancer (see the section on page 124 on "Choosing between lumpectomy and mastectomy").

Radiation therapy is sometimes omitted from breast-conserving therapy. Although this approach is somewhat controversial, women may consider lumpectomy without radiation therapy if they have all of the following characteristics:

- They are age 70 years or older.
- They have a tumor 2 cm or smaller that has been completely removed (with clear margins).
- They have a tumor that is hormone receptor–positive and are receiving hormone therapy (such as tamoxifen or an aromatase inhibitor).
- There is no lymph node involvement.

You should discuss this possibility with your health care team.

Possible side effects: Side effects of breast-conserving surgeries can include pain, temporary swelling, tenderness, and hard scar tissue that forms in the surgical site. As with all operations, bleeding and infection at the surgery site are also possible.

The larger the portion of breast removed, the more likely it is that there will be a noticeable change in the shape of the breast afterward. If the breast looks very different after surgery, it may be possible to have some type of reconstructive surgery (discussed later in this chapter) or to have the unaffected breast reduced in size to make the breasts more symmetrical. It may even be possible for these options to be done during the initial surgery. It is very important to talk with your doctor (and possibly a plastic surgeon) before surgery to get an idea of how your breasts are likely to look afterward and what options you may have.

Mastectomy

A mastectomy involves removing all of the breast tissue, sometimes along with other nearby tissues.

In a simple or **total mastectomy**, the surgeon removes the entire breast including the nipple, but does not remove axillary lymph nodes or muscle tissue from beneath the breast. In a double mastectomy, both breasts are removed. Sometimes this is done as preventive surgery for women at very high risk for breast cancer. Most women, if they are hospitalized, go home the next day.

For some women considering immediate reconstruction, a **skin-sparing mastectomy** can be done. In this procedure, most of the skin over the breast (other than the nipple and areola) is left intact. This can work as well as a simple mastectomy. The amount of breast tissue removed is the same as with a simple mastectomy. A skin-sparing mastectomy is used only when immediate breast reconstruction is planned. Implants or tissue from other parts of the body are then used to reconstruct the breast. Although this approach is newer than the more standard type of mastectomy, many women prefer it because it offers the advantage of less scar tissue and a reconstructed breast that seems more natural. A skin-sparing mastectomy may not be appropriate for larger tumors or those that are close to the skin.

A variation of the skin-sparing mastectomy is the **nipple-sparing mastectomy**. This procedure is more often an option for women who have a small, early-stage cancer near the outer part of the breast, with no signs of cancer in the skin or near the nipple. In this procedure, the breast tissue is removed, but the breast skin and nipple are left in place. This is followed by breast reconstruction. The surgeon often removes the breast tissue beneath the nipple (and areola) during the procedure, to check for cancer cells. If cancer is found in this tissue, the nipple is involved with cancer and must be removed. Even when no cancer is found under the nipple, some doctors give the nipple tissue a dose of radiation during or after the surgery to try and reduce the risk for cancer recurrence.

There are still some problems with nipple-sparing operations. After the procedure, the nipple will not have a good blood supply, so sometimes it can wither away or become deformed. Because the nerves are also cut, there is little or no feeling left in the nipple. In women with larger breasts, the nipple may look out of place after breast reconstruction. As a result, many doctors feel that the nipple-sparing operation is best restricted to women with small- to medium-sized breasts.

A nipple-sparing procedure is associated with less visible scars, but if the operation is not properly done, it can leave behind more breast tissue than other forms of mastectomy. This could result in a higher risk for cancer to recur, as compared with the risk associated with a skin-sparing or simple mastectomy. In recent years, however, improvements in technique have helped make this surgery safer. Still, many experts consider nipple-sparing procedures to be too risky for standard treatment of breast cancer.

A **modified radical mastectomy** involves removing the entire breast and some of the axillary lymph nodes. Surgery to remove these lymph nodes is discussed in further detail later in this section.

A **radical mastectomy** is an extensive operation in which the surgeon removes the entire breast, axillary lymph nodes, and the **pectoral** (chest wall) **muscles** under the breast. This surgery was once very common. However, a modified radical mastectomy has been proven to be as just as effective without the disfigurement and side effects of a radical mastectomy. Radical mastectomies are rarely done now. This operation may still be done for large tumors that are growing into the pectoral muscles under the breast.

Possible side effects: Aside from post-surgical pain and the obvious change in the shape of the breast(s), possible side effects of mastectomy include wound infection, **hematoma** (buildup of blood in the wound), and **seroma** (buildup of clear fluid in the wound). If axillary lymph nodes are also removed, other side effects may occur (see the section "Axillary lymph node dissection" on page 126).

Choosing between lumpectomy and mastectomy

Many women with early-stage breast cancer can choose between breast-conserving surgery and mastectomy. The main advantage of a lumpectomy is that it allows a woman to keep most of her breast. A disadvantage is the usual need for radiation therapy—most often for 5 to 6 weeks—after surgery. A small number of women having breast-conserving surgery may not need radiation (see the section on partial mastectomy), while a small percentage of women who have a mastectomy will still need radiation therapy to the breast area.

When deciding between a lumpectomy and a mastectomy, learn as much as possible about the procedures. Your initial gut reaction may be to choose mastectomy as a way to "take it all out as quickly as possible." This feeling can lead women to prefer mastectomy more often than their surgeons do. But the fact is that, in most cases, a mastectomy does not give you any better chance of long-term survival or a better outcome from treatment. Studies following thousands of women for more than 20 years show that in cases where a lumpectomy can be done, doing mastectomy instead does not provide any better chance of survival.

Although most women and their doctors prefer lumpectomy and radiation therapy when it is a reasonable option, your choice will depend on a number of factors:

- how you feel about losing your breast
- how you feel about receiving radiation therapy
- how far you would have to travel and how much time it would take to have radiation therapy
- whether you think you will want to have reconstructive surgery after a mastectomy
- your preference for mastectomy as a way to "get rid of all your cancer as quickly as possible"
- your fear of cancer recurrence

For some women, mastectomy may clearly be a better option. Lumpectomy or breast-conservation therapy is usually not recommended for women in the following situations:

- women who already have had radiation therapy to the affected breast
- women with 2 or more areas of cancer in the same breast that are too far apart to be removed through 1 surgical incision without significantly disturbing the appearance of the breast
- women for whom an initial lumpectomy and reexcision(s) have not completely removed the cancer
- women with serious connective tissue diseases such as scleroderma or lupus, which may make them more sensitive to the side effects of radiation therapy

- pregnant women who would require radiation while still pregnant (risking harm to the fetus)
- women with a tumor larger than 5 cm (2 inches) across that does not shrink very much with neoadjuvant chemotherapy
- women with inflammatory breast cancer
- women with tumors that are large relative to the breast size

Other factors may need to be taken into account as well. For example, young women with breast cancer and a known BRCA mutation are at very high risk for a second cancer. These women may want to consider having a mastectomy or a double mastectomy, both to treat the cancer and to reduce this risk.

Axillary lymph node dissection

To determine whether the breast cancer has spread to axillary (underarm) lymph nodes, some of these lymph nodes may be removed and examined under the microscope. This process is an important part of staging and determining treatment and outcomes. When lymph nodes are affected, there is an increased likelihood that cancer cells have spread through the bloodstream to other parts of the body.

As noted earlier, **axillary lymph node dissection (ALND)** is part of a radical or modified radical mastectomy. It may also be done as part of a breast-conserving procedure such as lumpectomy. Anywhere from about 10 to 40 (though usually less than 20) lymph nodes are removed. The presence of cancer cells in the lymph nodes under the arm is an important factor in considering adjuvant therapy. Axillary dissection is used as a test to help guide other breast cancer treatment decisions.

Possible side effects: The main possible long-term effect of removing axillary lymph nodes is lymphedema (swelling of the arm). This swelling occurs because excess fluid in the arms normally travels back into the bloodstream through the lymphatic system. Removing the lymph nodes sometimes blocks the drainage from the arm, causing this fluid to remain and build up in the arm.

Up to 30% of women who have axillary lymph nodes removed develop lymphedema. It also occurs in up to 3% of women who have a sentinel lymph node biopsy (discussed on page 128). It may be more common if radiation is given after surgery. Sometimes the swelling lasts for only a few weeks and then goes away. Other times, the swelling lasts a long time. Lymphedema is a chronic condition. It can be managed but is not curable. Efforts can be made to reduce your risk.

Ways to help prevent or reduce the effects of lymphedema are discussed in the section "What Happens After Treatment for Breast Cancer?" on pages 209–211. If your arm is swollen, tight, or painful after lymph node surgery, tell someone on your cancer care team right away.

As with other operations, pain, swelling, bleeding, and infection are possible. You may also have short- or long-term limitations in moving your arm and shoulder after surgery. Your doctor may give you exercises to ensure that you do not have permanent problems with movement, such as a frozen shoulder. Numbness of the skin of the upper inner arm is another common side effect of axillary lymph node dissection because the nerve that controls sensation there travels through the lymph node area.

Sentinel lymph node biopsy

Although axillary lymph node dissection is a safe operation with low rates of most side effects other than lymphedema, in many cases doctors will first choose a **sentinel lymph node biopsy (SLNB)** to check the lymph nodes for cancer. This type of biopsy can show whether cancer has spread to lymph nodes without removing all of them.

In this procedure, the surgeon finds and removes the first lymph node(s) into which a tumor drains. This lymph node, known as the sentinel node, is the one most likely to contain cancer cells if they have spread. To do this, the surgeon injects a radioactive substance and/or a blue dye into the tumor or the area around it. Lymphatic vessels will carry the substance(s) into the sentinel node(s). The doctor then uses a special device to detect the lymph nodes that have attracted the radioactive solution or to look for lymph nodes that have turned blue. These are separate ways to find the sentinel node, but they are often done together as a safeguard. The doctor then cuts the skin over the area and removes the nodes containing the dye (or radiation). These nodes (often 2 or 3) are then examined by the pathologist. (Because fewer nodes are removed than with an axillary lymph node dissection, each one can be studied very closely for any cancer).

If there is no cancer in the sentinel node(s), it is very unlikely that the cancer has spread to other lymph nodes. Therefore, no further lymph node surgery is needed. The person can avoid the potential side effects of an axillary lymph node dissection.

If cancer cells are found in the sentinel node(s), the surgeon will perform an axillary lymph node dissection to see how many other lymph nodes are involved. The sentinel lymph node(s) can sometimes be checked for cancer during the breast surgery. If cancer is found in the sentinel lymph node, the surgeon may go on to remove more lymph nodes or even perform an axillary dissection at that time. If no cancer cells can be seen in the lymph node during surgery, or if the sentinel node is not checked during surgery, the lymph node(s) will be examined in greater detail over the next several days. If cancer is found in the lymph node, the surgeon may recommend an axillary lymph node dissection at a later time.

Sentinel lymph node biopsy requires a great deal of skill. It should be done only by a surgical team known to have experience with this technique. If you are thinking about having this type of biopsy, ask your cancer care team if they perform it regularly.

Possible side effects: As with other operations, pain, swelling, bleeding, and infection are possible.

The main possible long-term effect of a sentinel lymph node biopsy is lymphedema of the arm. This occurs less often with this procedure than with a full axillary lymph node dissection, but it can still happen. Lymphedema is discussed in more detail in the previous section on axillary lymph node dissection and on page 209.

Reconstructive surgery

After having a mastectomy (or some breast-conserving surgeries), some women consider having the breast rebuilt. This procedure is called **breast reconstruction**. Breast reconstruction is not done to treat cancer but to restore the appearance of the breast after surgery. If you are going to have breast surgery and are thinking about having reconstruction, it is important to consult with a plastic surgeon who is an expert in breast reconstruction before your surgery. For more information on breast reconstruction, see pages 188–203.

What to expect with surgery

For many women, the thought of surgery can be frightening. However, many fears can be relieved with a better understanding of what to expect before, during, and after the operation.

Before surgery: You will be contacted within a few days of most common biopsy procedures if you have breast cancer. However, the extent of the breast cancer will not be known until after imaging tests and the surgery for local treatment are completed. Most likely, you will meet with your surgeon a few days before the operation to discuss the procedure. This is a good time to ask specific questions about the surgery and review potential risks. Be sure you understand the extent of the surgery and what you should expect afterward. If you are thinking about breast reconstruction, this meeting is a good time to ask about this as well.

You will be asked to sign a consent form giving the doctor permission to perform the surgery. Take your time and review the form carefully to be certain that you understand what you are signing. Sometimes doctors send material for you to review in advance of your appointment so that you have plenty of time to read it without feeling rushed. You may also be asked to give consent for researchers to use any tissue or blood that is not needed for diagnostic purposes. Although giving your consent may not benefit you directly, it may be useful in research that will help other women in the future.

You may be asked to donate blood before the operation if the doctors think a transfusion might be needed. You might feel more secure in knowing that if a transfusion is needed, you will receive your own blood. If you do not receive your own blood, it is important to know that in the United States, a blood transfusion from another person is nearly as safe as receiving your own blood. Ask your doctor about your possible need for a blood transfusion.

Your doctor will review your medical records and ask you about any medicines you are taking to be sure you are not taking anything that could interfere with the surgery. For example, if you are taking aspirin, arthritis medicine, or a blood-thinning drug (such as coumadin), you may need to stop taking the drug for a brief period before the surgery. Tell your doctor about any medications or supplements you take, including vitamins and herbal supplements. You will probably be told not to eat or drink anything for 8 to 12 hours before the surgery, especially if you are going to have general anesthesia (you will be "asleep" during surgery).

You will also meet with the anesthesiologist or nurse anesthetist, the health care professional who will administer your anesthesia during the surgery. The type of anesthesia used depends largely on the kind of surgery being done and your medical history.

During surgery: Depending on the extent of your surgery, you may be offered the choice of an outpatient procedure (where you go home the same day) or you may be admitted to the hospital.

General anesthesia is usually given when surgery involves a mastectomy or an axillary lymph node dissection, and it is most often used during breast-conserving surgery as well. An intravenous (IV) line will be put in (usually in your arm), which the medical team will use to give any medicines that are needed during surgery. You will probably be hooked up to an electrocardiogram (EKG) machine and have a blood pressure cuff on your arm so that your heart rhythm and blood pressure can be monitored during surgery.

The length of the operation depends on the type of surgery. For example, a mastectomy with axillary lymph node dissection will usually take from 2 to 3 hours. After your surgery, you will be taken to the recovery room, where you will remain until you are awake and your condition and vital signs (blood pressure, pulse, and breathing) are stable.

After surgery: The length of your stay in the hospital depends on the type of surgery, your overall health and whether you have any other medical problems, how well you do during the surgery, and how you feel after the surgery. Decisions about the length of your stay should be made by you and your doctor and not dictated by what your insurance will pay. However, it is important to check your insurance coverage before surgery. In general, women having a mastectomy and/or axillary lymph node dissection are hospitalized for 1 or 2 nights. Some women may be placed in a 23-hour, short-stay observation unit before going home. Less involved operations, such as lumpectomy and sentinel lymph node biopsy, are often done in an outpatient surgery center, and an overnight stay in the hospital is usually not needed.

You may have a dressing (bandage) over the surgery site, which may wrap snugly around your chest. You may also have one or more drains (plastic or rubber tubes) coming out of the breast or underarm area to remove blood and lymph fluid that collects during the healing process. Your cancer care team will teach you how to care for the drains. This may include emptying and measuring the fluid and identifying problems that need to be shared with the doctor or nurse. Most drains stay in place for 1 or 2 weeks. When drainage has decreased to about 30 cc (1 fluid ounce) each day, the drain will usually be removed. Most doctors will want you to start moving your arm soon after surgery so that it will not become stiff.

Many women who have a lumpectomy or mastectomy are surprised by how little pain they have in the breast area. But they are often bothered by the strange sensations (such as numbness and pinching or pulling feelings) they may feel in the underarm area.

Ask your cancer care team how to care for your surgery site and arm. They will probably give you and your caregivers written instructions about care after surgery that should include the following:

- how to care for the surgical wound and dressing
- how to monitor drainage and take care of the drains
- how to recognize signs of infection
- when to call the doctor or nurse
- when to begin using your arm and how to do arm exercises to prevent stiffness
- when to resume wearing a bra
- when to begin using a prosthesis and what type to use (after a mastectomy)
- what to eat and what foods to avoid
- what medications to take, including pain medicines and possibly antibiotics
- any restrictions on activity
- what to expect regarding sensations or numbness in the breast and arm
- what to expect regarding feelings about body image

- when to see your doctor for a follow-up appointment
- how to be referred to a Reach to Recovery volunteer

Most patients see their doctor about 7 to 14 days after the surgery. Your doctor will explain the results of your pathology report and talk to you about the need for further treatment. If more treatment is needed, you may be referred to a radiation oncologist and/or a medical oncologist. If you are thinking about breast reconstruction, you may be referred to a plastic surgeon as well.

Post-mastectomy pain syndrome

Post-mastectomy pain syndrome (PMPS) is chronic neuropathic (nerve) pain that occurs after lumpectomy or mastectomy. Studies have shown that PMPS occurs in 20% and 60% of women who have a lumpectomy or mastectomy, but it is often not recognized as such. The classic signs of PMPS are pain in the chest wall and tingling down the arm. Pain may also be felt in the shoulder, scar, arm, or armpit. Other common complaints include numbness, shooting or pricking pain, or unbearable itching. PMPS is thought to be linked to damage done to the nerves in the underarm and chest during surgery, but the causes are not known. Because major surgeries are used less frequently to treat breast cancer today, PMPS is becoming less of a problem.

It is important to talk to your doctor about any pain you are having. PMPS can prevent you from using your arm the way you should and, over time, you could lose the ability to use it normally. PMPS can be treated. Opioids or narcotics are commonly used to treat pain, but they don't always work well for nerve pain. There are medicines and treatments that do work for this kind of pain. Talk to your doctor to get the pain control you need.

Radiation Therapy

Radiation therapy is treatment with high-energy rays or particles that destroy cancer cells. This treatment may be used to kill any cancer cells that remain in the breast, chest wall, or underarm area after breast-conserving surgery. Radiation may also be needed after a mastectomy in cases in which the tumor is 5 cm in size or larger or when cancer is found in the lymph nodes.

Radiation therapy can be given in 2 main ways: external beam radiation therapy and brachy-therapy.

External beam radiation therapy

External beam radiation therapy is the most common type of radiation therapy for women with breast cancer. The radiation is focused from a machine outside the body on the area affected by the cancer.

The extent of radiation depends on whether a lumpectomy or mastectomy was done and whether lymph nodes are involved. If a lumpectomy was done, most often the entire breast receives radiation, and an extra boost of radiation is given to the area where the cancer was removed to prevent recurrence in that area. Depending on the size and extent of the cancer, the radiation treatment area may include the chest wall and underarm area. In some cases, the treatment area may also include supraclavicular lymph nodes (nodes above the collarbone) and internal mammary lymph nodes (nodes beneath the breastbone in the center of the chest).

When given after surgery, external beam radiation therapy is usually not started until the tissues have healed, often a month or longer. If chemotherapy is to be given as well, radiation therapy is usually delayed until chemotherapy is complete.

Before your treatments start, the radiation team will take careful measurements to determine the correct angles for aiming the radiation beams and the proper dose of radiation. They will make ink marks or small tattoos on your skin that will be used later as guides to focus the radiation on the correct area. You may want to talk to your health care team to find out whether these marks will be permanent. Lotions, powders, deodorants, and antiperspirants can interfere with external beam radiation therapy, so your cancer care team may tell you not to use these products until treatments are complete.

External radiation therapy is much like getting an x-ray, but the radiation is more intense. The procedure itself is painless. Each treatment lasts only a few minutes, although the setup time—getting you into place for treatment—usually takes longer.

The most common treatment schedule for a woman receiving breast radiation is 5 days a week (Monday through Friday) for about 5 to 6 weeks.

Accelerated breast irradiation: The standard treatment schedule, in which a woman receives external radiation for 5 days a week over many weeks, can be inconvenient for many women. Some doctors are now using other schedules, such as giving slightly larger daily doses over a period of only 3 weeks. This approach was studied in a large group of women who had been treated with breast-conserving surgery and did not have cancer spread to underarm lymph nodes. When compared with giving the radiation over 5 weeks, giving it over only 3 weeks worked just as well in keeping the cancer from recurring in the same breast during the first 10 years after treatment. Giving radiation in larger doses using fewer treatments is known as hypofractionated radiation therapy. Newer approaches now being studied shorten the treatment period even more. In one approach, larger doses of radiation are given each day, but the course of radiation is shortened to only 5 days. In another approach, known as **intraoperative radiation therapy (IORT)**, a single large dose of radiation is given in the operating room right after a lumpectomy (before the breast incision is closed).

Other forms of **accelerated breast irradiation** are described below in the section on brachytherapy. It is hoped that these newer approaches will prove to be at least equal to the current, standard approach to radiation therapy for breast cancer, but few studies have been done comparing these new methods directly to standard radiation therapy. It is not known whether all of the newer methods will still be as good as standard radiation after many years. For this reason, many doctors still consider them experimental. Women who are interested in these approaches may want to ask their doctor about taking part in clinical trials of accelerated breast irradiation.

3D-conformal radiotherapy: With 3D-conformal radiotherapy, the radiation is given using special machines so that the radiation is more precisely aimed at the cancerous area. This allows more of the healthy breast to be spared. Treatments are given twice a day for 5 days. Because only part of the breast is treated, this is considered to be a form of accelerated partial breast irradiation.

Possible side effects of external beam radiation therapy: The main short-term side effects of external beam radiation therapy are swelling and heaviness in the breast, sunburn-like skin changes in the treated area, and **fatigue**. Your health care team may advise you to avoid exposing the treated skin to the sun because it may make the skin changes worse. Changes to the breast tissue and skin usually go away in 6 to 12 months.

In some women, the breast becomes smaller and firmer after radiation therapy. Because of these changes, receiving radiation therapy may also affect a woman's chances of having breast reconstruction. Women who have had breast radiation may also have later problems with breastfeeding. Radiation to the breast can sometimes damage some of the nerves to the arm. This effect, known as **brachial plexopathy**, can lead to numbness, pain, and weakness in the shoulder, arm, and hand.

Radiation therapy of axillary lymph nodes also can cause lymphedema (see the section "What Happens After Treatment for Breast Cancer?" on pages 209–211). In rare cases, radiation therapy can weaken the ribs, which could lead to a fracture. In the past, parts of the lungs and heart were more likely to be exposed to radiation, which could lead to long-term damage of these organs. Modern radiation therapy equipment allows doctors to better focus the radiation beams, so these problems are rare today.

A very rare complication of radiation to the breast is the development of another cancer called angiosarcoma (see "What Is Breast Cancer?" on page 15). These rare cancers can grow and spread quickly.

Brachytherapy

Brachytherapy, also known as internal radiation, is another way to deliver radiation therapy. Instead of aiming radiation beams from outside the body, radioactive seeds or pellets are placed directly into the breast tissue next to the cancer. This treatment is often used as a way to add an extra boost of radiation to the tumor site along with external radiation to the whole breast, although it may also be used by itself. Tumor size, location, and other factors may limit who can receive brachytherapy. There are several different types of brachytherapy.

Intracavitary brachytherapy: Intracavitary brachytherapy consists of a small balloon attached to a thin tube. The deflated balloon is inserted into the space left by the lumpectomy and is filled with a salt water solution. (This can be done at the time of the lumpectomy or up to several weeks afterward.) The balloon and tube are left in place throughout the treatment (with the end of the tube sticking out of the breast). Twice a day, a source of radioactivity is placed into the middle of the balloon through the tube and then removed. This is done for 5 days as an outpatient treatment. The balloon is then deflated and removed. This system goes by the brand name Mammosite. This type of brachytherapy can also be considered a form of accelerated partial breast irradiation. Like many forms of accelerated breast irradiation, there are no studies comparing the outcomes for this type of radiation with standard external beam radiation. It is not known whether long-term outcomes will be as good.

Interstitial brachytherapy: With interstitial brachytherapy, several small catheters (hollow tubes) are inserted into the breast around the area of the lumpectomy and are left in place for several days. Radioactive pellets are inserted into the catheters for short periods of time each day and then removed. This method of brachytherapy has been around longer and has more evidence to support it, but it is not used as much anymore.

Brachytherapy is also being studied in clinical trials as the only source of radiation for women who have had a lumpectomy. In this sense, brachytherapy can also be considered a form of accelerated partial breast irradiation. Early results have been promising, but long-term results are not available. It is not yet clear whether irradiating only the area around the cancer will reduce the chances of recurrence as much as radiation to the whole breast. The results of studies now under way will probably be needed before more doctors recommend accelerated partial breast irradiation as a standard treatment option.

Chemotherapy

Chemotherapy (chemo) is treatment with cancer-killing drugs that are given intravenously (injected into a vein) or by mouth. It is a type of systemic therapy, meaning the drugs travel through the bloodstream to reach cancer cells throughout the body. Chemotherapy is given in cycles, with each treatment period followed by a recovery period. Treatment usually lasts for several months.

When chemotherapy is used

There are several situations in which chemotherapy may be recommended.

Adjuvant chemotherapy: Systemic therapy given to patients who have no evidence of cancer after surgery is called adjuvant therapy. Whereas surgery is used to remove the cancer that can be seen, adjuvant therapy is used to kill any cancer cells that may have been left behind but cannot be seen. When used as adjuvant therapy after breast-conserving surgery or mastectomy, chemotherapy reduces the risk for breast cancer recurrence. Both chemotherapy and hormone therapy can be used as adjuvant therapies.

Even in the early stages of the disease, cancer cells may break away from the primary tumor and spread through the bloodstream. These cells do not cause symptoms, do not show up on imaging tests, and cannot be detected during a physical examination. But if allowed to grow, they can establish new tumors in other places in the body. The goal of adjuvant chemotherapy is to kill undetected cells that have traveled from the breast.

Neoadjuvant chemotherapy: Chemotherapy given before surgery is called neoadjuvant therapy. Neoadjuvant therapy often uses the same chemotherapy drugs used in adjuvant therapy (only before surgery instead of after). In terms of survival, there is no difference between giving chemotherapy before or after surgery. The major benefit of neoadjuvant chemotherapy is that it can shrink large cancers so that they are small enough to be removed by lumpectomy instead of mastectomy. Another possible advantage of neoadjuvant chemotherapy is that doctors can see how the cancer responds to chemotherapy. If the tumor does not shrink, your doctor may try different chemotherapy drugs.

Chemotherapy for advanced breast cancer: Chemotherapy can also be used as the main treatment for women whose cancer has spread outside the breast and underarm area at the time of diagnosis or whose cancer spreads after initial treatments. The length of treatment depends on whether the cancer shrinks, how much it shrinks, and how the woman tolerates treatment.

How chemotherapy is administered

In most cases (especially for adjuvant and neoadjuvant treatment), chemotherapy is most effective when combinations of more than one drug are used. Many different combinations are used, but it is unclear whether any single combination is the best. Clinical studies continue to compare today's most effective treatments against newer combinations that may be more effective.

These are some of the most commonly used drug combinations:

- CMF: cyclophosphamide (Cytoxan), methotrexate, and 5-fluorouracil (fluorouracil, 5-FU)
- CAF (FAC): cyclophosphamide, doxorubicin (Adriamycin), and 5-fluorouracil
- AC: doxorubicin and cyclophosphamide
- EC: epirubicin (Ellence) and cyclophosphamide
- TAC: docetaxel (Taxotere), doxorubicin, and cyclophosphamide
- AC → T: doxorubicin and cyclophosphamide, followed by paclitaxel (Taxol) or docetaxel. (Trastuzumab [Herceptin] may be given with the paclitaxel or docetaxel for HER2/neu positive tumors.)
- A → CMF: doxorubicin, followed by CMF
- CEF (FEC): cyclophosphamide, epirubicin, and 5-fluorouracil (this may be followed by docetaxel)
- TC: docetaxel and cyclophosphamide
- TCH: docetaxel, carboplatin, and trastuzumab for HER2/neu positive tumors

Other chemotherapy drugs used for treating women with breast cancer include cisplatin, vinorelbine (Navelbine), capecitabine (Xeloda), pegylated liposomal doxorubicin (Doxil), gemcitibine (Gemzar), mitoxantrone, ixabepilone (Ixempra), and albumin-bound paclitaxel (Abraxane). The targeted therapy drugs trastuzumab and lapatinib (Tykerb) may be used with these chemotherapy drugs for tumors that are HER2/neu-positive (these drugs are discussed in more detail in the "Targeted Therapy" section on pages 156–159).

Doctors give chemotherapy in cycles, with each treatment period followed by a recovery period. The chemotherapy begins on the first day of each cycle, and then the body is given time to recover from the effects of chemotherapy. The chemotherapy drugs are then repeated to start the next cycle. The period between receiving the chemotherapy drugs is generally 2 or 3 weeks and varies according to the specific drug or combination of drugs. Some drugs are given more frequently. The treatment cycle generally lasts for a total period of 3 to 6 months when given after surgery, depending on the drugs used. Treatment may be longer for advanced breast cancer.

Dose-dense chemotherapy: Doctors have found that shortening the time between chemotherapy doses—an approach called dose-dense chemotherapy—can lower the chance of recurrence and improve survival in some women. With this approach, the woman would usually receive chemotherapy every 2 weeks instead of every 3 weeks (such as AC → T). In addition, a drug called a growth factor is given after the chemotherapy to help the white blood cell count return to normal in time for the next cycle. Dose-dense chemotherapy can lead to more side effects and be harder to endure, so it is only used for treatment in women who are at high risk for recurrence.

Possible side effects of chemotherapy

Chemotherapy drugs work by attacking cells that divide quickly, which is why they work against cancer cells. But other cells in the body also divide quickly, such as those in the **bone marrow**, the lining of the mouth and intestines, and the hair follicles. These cells are also likely to be affected by chemotherapy, which can lead to side effects. Some women have many side effects whereas other women experience few side effects.

The side effects of chemotherapy depend on the type of drugs, the amount taken, and the length of treatment. These are some of the most common possible side effects:

- hair loss
- mouth sores
- loss of appetite
- nausea and vomiting
- increased chance of infections (due to low **white blood cell** counts)
- easy bruising or bleeding (due to low blood platelet counts)
- fatigue (due to low **red blood cell** counts and other reasons)

These side effects usually do not last long and go away after treatment is finished. It is important to let your health care team know if you have any side effects, as there are often ways to lessen their intensity. For example, drugs can be given to help prevent or reduce nausea and vomiting.

Several other side effects are also possible. Some of these are only seen with certain chemotherapy drugs. Your cancer care team will give you information about the possible side effects of the specific drugs you are taking.

Menstrual changes: For younger women, changes in menstrual periods are a common side effect of chemotherapy. Premature menopause (not having any more menstrual periods) and infertility (not being able to become pregnant) are possible permanent complications of chemotherapy. Some chemotherapy drugs are more likely to have these side effects than others. The older a woman is when she undergoes chemotherapy, the more likely it is that she will become infertile or menopausal as a result. These side effects can also lead to rapid bone loss from osteoporosis. Again, there are medicines that can treat or help prevent problems with bone loss.

You cannot assume that chemotherapy will prevent pregnancy, and getting pregnant while undergoing chemotherapy can lead to birth defects and interfere with treatment. For this reason, premenopausal women who are sexually active should discuss their options for birth control with their doctor. It is safe to have children after chemotherapy (if it is still possible for the individual woman), but it is not safe to get pregnant while undergoing treatment. If you are pregnant when your breast cancer is diagnosed, you still can be treated. Chemotherapy can be given safely during the last 2 trimesters of pregnancy.

Neuropathy: Neuropathy is a condition that affects certain nerves in the body. It causes numbness and other sensations in certain parts of the body, especially the hands and feet. Several drugs used to treat breast cancer—including the taxanes (docetaxel and paclitaxel), platinum agents (carboplatin, cisplatin), and ixabepilone—can damage nerves outside of the brain and spinal cord. This damage can sometimes lead to symptoms (mainly in the hands and feet) such as numbness, pain, burning or tingling sensations, sensitivity to cold or heat, or weakness. In most cases, this side effect goes away once treatment ends, but it may last longer in some women.

Heart damage: Doxorubicin, epirubicin, and some other drugs may cause permanent heart damage if administered in high doses or used for an extended time. For this reason, doctors often check the patient's heart function before starting one of these drugs. They also carefully control the doses and use echocardiograms or other tests to monitor heart function. If the person's heart function begins to decline, treatment with these drugs will be stopped. In some patients, however, heart damage can take a long time to develop, and they may show signs of poor heart function months or years later. Heart damage from these drugs happens more often if the targeted therapy drug trastuzumab is used as well, so doctors are more cautious when these drugs are used together.

Hand-foot syndrome: Certain chemotherapy drugs, such as capecitabine and liposomal doxorubicin, can cause problems with irritation that affects the palms of the hands and the soles of the feet. This is called hand-foot syndrome. Early symptoms include numbness, tingling, and redness. If it gets worse, the hands and feet become swollen with discomfort or even pain. The skin may blister, leading to peeling of the skin. There is no specific treatment, but these symptoms gradually get better when the drug is stopped. The best way to prevent severe hand-foot syndrome is to tell your doctor when early symptoms come up, so that the drug dosage can be changed. Hand-foot syndrome can also occur when the drug 5-FU is given as an intravenous infusion over several days (which is not common in the treatment of breast cancer).

Chemo brain: Many women who undergo chemotherapy for breast cancer report a slight decrease in mental functioning, a side effect known as "chemo brain." Some women have problems with concentration and memory, which may last a long time. Still, most women function well after chemotherapy. The symptoms usually go away within a few years. For more information, contact your American Cancer Society at **800-227-2345** and request the document *Chemo Brain,* or visit our Web site, **cancer.org**.

Increased risk of leukemia: Very rarely, certain chemotherapy drugs can permanently damage the bone marrow, leading to acute myeloid leukemia, a life-threatening cancer of the white blood cells.

When this happens, it usually occurs within 10 years of treatment. In most women, the benefits of chemotherapy in preventing breast cancer recurrence or in extending life far exceed the risk for this serious but rare complication.

Feeling unwell or tired: Many women do not feel as healthy after receiving chemotherapy as they did before starting treatment. Many women have residual body pains or achiness and a mild loss of physical functioning. The changes are usually very subtle, and some women may not notice such a change.

Fatigue is another common (but often overlooked) problem for women who have received chemotherapy. This condition may last for several years. It can often be helped, so it is important to discuss this side effect with your doctor or nurse. Exercise, naps, and taking steps to conserve energy may be recommended. If there are sleep problems, these can be treated. Sometimes the fatigue is accompanied by depression, which may be helped by counseling and/or medicines. For more information on what you can do to cope with fatigue, contact your American Cancer Society at **800-227-2345** and request the document *Fatigue in People with Cancer,* or visit our Web site, **cancer.org**.

Hormone Therapy

Hormone therapy is another form of systemic therapy. It is most often used as an adjuvant therapy to help reduce the risk of cancer recurrence after surgery, although it can also be used as neoadjuvant treatment. Hormone therapy is also used to treat cancer that has come back after treatment or cancer that has spread. It can be used in combination with a number of different types of treatments.

A woman's ovaries are the main source of the hormone estrogen until menopause. After menopause, smaller amounts are still made in the body's fat tissue, where a hormone made by the adrenal gland is converted into estrogen.

Estrogen promotes the growth of about 2 of every 3 of breast cancers—those containing estrogen receptors (ER–positive cancers) and/or progesterone receptors (PR–positive cancers). Several approaches to blocking the effect of estrogen or lowering estrogen levels are used to treat ER–positive and PR–positive breast cancers. Hormone therapy does not help patients whose tumors are not ER– or PR–positive.

Tamoxifen and toremifene

Tamoxifen (Nolvadex) and toremifene (Fareston) are antiestrogen drugs that work by temporarily blocking estrogen receptors on breast cancer cells, preventing estrogen from binding to them. They are taken daily in pill form.

For women with hormone receptor–positive cancers, taking tamoxifen after surgery for 5 years reduces the chances of cancer recurrence by about half. Tamoxifen can also be used to treat metastatic breast cancer (cancer that has spread from the breast to other parts of the body) and to reduce the risk of breast cancer in women who are at high risk. Toremifene works like tamoxifen, but it is not used as often.

The most common side effects of tamoxifen and toremifene include fatigue, hot flashes, vaginal dryness or discharge, and mood swings. Some patients whose cancer has spread to their bones (bone metastasis) may experience a "tumor flare" and have pain and swelling in the muscles and bones. This reaction usually subsides quickly, but in some cases these patients can also develop a high calcium level in the blood that cannot be controlled. If this occurs, the treatment may need to be stopped.

Rare, but more serious side effects of antiestrogen drugs are also possible. These drugs can increase the risk of developing cancers of the uterus (endometrial cancer and uterine sarcoma). Tell your doctor right away about any unusual vaginal bleeding (a common symptom of both of these cancers). Most vaginal bleeding is not from cancer, but this symptom always needs prompt attention.

Another possible serious side effect of antiestrogen drugs is a blood clot, which usually forms in the legs. In some cases, blood clots can lead to a heart attack, stroke, or blockage in the lungs (pulmonary embolism). Contact your doctor or nurse immediately if you develop pain, redness, or swelling in your lower leg, shortness of breath, chest pain, sudden severe headache, confusion, or have trouble speaking or moving.

The effects of tamoxifen on the bones can vary, depending on the woman's menopausal status. In premenopausal women, tamoxifen can cause some bone thinning. However, in postmenopausal women, tamoxifen is often beneficial for bone strength. The effects of toremifene on the bones are less clear.

For most women with breast cancer, the benefits of taking these drugs outweigh the risks.

Fulvestrant

Fulvestrant (Faslodex) is a drug that also acts on the estrogen receptor. But instead of blocking the estrogen receptor, this drug eliminates it. It is often effective even if the breast cancer is no longer responding to tamoxifen. Fulvestrant is given by injection once a month. Hot flashes, mild nausea, and fatigue are the major side effects. It is currently only approved for use in postmenopausal women with advanced breast cancer that is no longer responding to tamoxifen or toremifene.

Aromatase inhibitors

Three drugs that stop estrogen production in postmenopausal women have been approved to treat both early-stage and advanced breast cancer: letrozole (Femara), anastrozole (Arimidex), and exemestane (Aromasin). These drugs work by blocking aromatase, an enzyme that is responsible for making small amounts of estrogen in postmenopausal women. Aromatase inhibitors cannot stop the ovaries of premenopausal women from making estrogen, so they are only effective in postmenopausal women. These drugs are taken daily in pill form.

Several studies have compared aromatase inhibitors with tamoxifen as adjuvant hormone therapy in postmenopausal women. Using these drugs, either alone or after tamoxifen, has been shown to better reduce the risk of cancer recurrence compared with using tamoxifen alone for 5 years.

These schedules are known to be helpful:

- tamoxifen for 2 to 3 years, followed by an aromatase inhibitor to complete 5 years of treatment
- tamoxifen for 5 years, followed by an aromatase inhibitor for 5 years
- an aromatase inhibitor for 5 years

Most doctors now recommend an aromatase inhibitor be administered at some point during adjuvant therapy in post-menopausal women with hormone receptor–positive cancers. But it is unclear whether starting adjuvant therapy with one of these drugs is better than prescribing tamoxifen and then switching to an aromatase inhibitor. We still don't know whether giving these drugs for more than 5 years is more helpful than stopping at 5 years. It is also unknown whether any one of these drugs is better than the others. Studies are now under way to address these questions.

Aromatase inhibitors tend to have fewer serious side effects than tamoxifen—they don't cause uterine cancers and very rarely cause blood clots. They can, however, cause muscle pain and joint stiffness and/or pain. The joint pain may be similar to a new feeling of having arthritis in many different joints at one time. Although joint pain may improve by switching to a different aromatase inhibitor, this side effect has prompted some women to stop drug treatment. If this occurs, most doctors recommend using tamoxifen to complete 5 years of hormone treatment.

Because aromatase inhibitors remove all estrogen in postmenopausal women, they also cause bone thinning, sometimes leading to osteoporosis or even fractures. Many women treated with an aromatase inhibitor are also treated with medicine to strengthen their bones, such as bisphosphonates.

Ovarian ablation

In premenopausal women, removing or shutting down the ovaries, which are the main source of estrogens, effectively makes the woman postmenopausal. This process is called **ovarian ablation**. This procedure may allow some other hormone therapies to work better.

Permanent ovarian ablation can be done by surgically removing the ovaries. This operation is called an **oophorectomy**. More often, ovarian ablation is done with drugs called luteinizing hormone-releasing hormone (LHRH) analogs, such as goserelin (Zoladex) or leuprolide (Lupron). These drugs stop the signal that the body sends to the ovaries to make estrogen. They can be used alone or with tamoxifen as hormone therapy in premenopausal women. They are also being studied as as a form of adjuvant therapy when combined with aromatase inhibitors in premenopausal women.

Chemotherapy drugs may also damage the ovaries of premenopausal women to the extent that the ovaries no longer produce estrogen. In some women, ovarian function returns months or years later, but in others, the damage to the ovaries is permanent and leads to menopause. This can sometimes be a helpful (if unintended) consequence of chemotherapy with regard to breast cancer treatment, although it leaves the woman infertile.

All methods of ovarian ablation can cause a woman to have symptoms of menopause, including hot flashes, night sweats, vaginal dryness, and mood swings.

Megestrol acetate

Megestrol acetate (Megace) is a progesterone-like drug used as a hormone treatment for advanced breast cancer, usually for women whose cancers have not responded to other hormone treatments. Its major side effect is weight gain, and it is sometimes used in higher doses to reverse weight loss in patients with advanced cancer. It is an older drug and is no longer used very often.

Other ways to control hormones

Androgens (male hormones) may be another option after other hormonal treatments for advanced breast cancer have been tried. Androgens are sometimes effective, but they can cause masculine characteristics such as an increase in body hair and development of a deeper voice.

Targeted Therapy

As researchers have learned more about the gene changes in cells that cause cancer, they have been able to develop newer drugs that specifically target these changes. These targeted drugs work differently from standard chemotherapy drugs. They often have different (and less severe) side effects. Targeted therapy is most often used with chemotherapy at this time.

Drugs that target the HER2/neu protein

Trastuzumab: Trastuzumab is a type of drug known as a **monoclonal antibody**—a man-made version of a very specific immune system protein. It attaches to a growth-promoting protein known as HER2/neu (or just HER2), which is present in larger than normal amounts on the surface of breast cancer cells in about 1 of 5 patients. Breast cancers with too much of this protein tend to grow and spread more aggressively. Trastuzumab can help slow this growth and may also stimulate the immune system to attack the cancer more effectively. Trastuzumab is given as an injection into a vein, usually once a week or in a larger dose every 3 weeks. The optimal length of time to give this drug has not yet been determined.

Trastuzumab is often used with chemotherapy as adjuvant therapy for HER2-positive cancers to reduce the risk of recurrence when the tumor is larger than 1 cm or there is lymph node involvement. It is given with chemotherapy for 3 to 6 months, and then given on its own, usually for a total treatment period of a year. Studies are under way looking at how long this drug needs to be given.

Trastuzumab can also shrink some HER2-positive advanced breast cancers that return after chemotherapy or that continue to grow during chemotherapy. Treatment that combines trastuzumab with chemotherapy may work better than chemotherapy alone in some patients.

Compared with chemotherapy drugs, the side effects of trastuzumab are relatively mild. They may include fever and chills, weakness, nausea, vomiting, cough, diarrhea, and headache. These side effects occur less often after the first dose.

A more serious potential side effect of trastuzumab is heart damage that leads to congestive heart failure. For most women, this effect is temporary and improves when the drug is stopped. The risk of heart problems is higher when trastuzumab is given with certain chemotherapy drugs such as doxorubicin and epirubicin. Symptoms of congestive heart failure include shortness of breath, leg swelling, and severe fatigue. Women experiencing these symptoms should call their doctors immediately.

Lapatinib: Lapatinib is another drug that targets the HER2 protein. This drug is given in pill form to women with advanced HER2-positive breast cancer that is no longer responding to chemotherapy and trastuzumab. Lapatinib is also being studied as an adjuvant therapy in HER2-positive patients, but at this time it is only used for advanced breast cancer. Women with advanced breast cancer who were given lapatinib along with trastuzumab lived longer than those who were given lapatinib alone. Capecitabine is often given as well.

The most common side effects of lapatinib include diarrhea, nausea, vomiting, rash, and hand-foot syndrome. Diarrhea is a common side effect and can be severe, so it is very important to contact your health care team immediately if you experience any changes in bowel habits. In rare cases, lapatinib can cause liver problems or a decrease in heart function that can lead to shortness of breath, although these side effects seem to go away once treatment is finished.

Drugs that target new tumor blood vessels

In order to grow, tumors need to develop and maintain new blood vessels (a process called **angiogenesis**). Drugs that target these blood vessels are proving to be helpful against a variety of cancers, including breast cancer.

Bevacizumab (Avastin) is a monoclonal antibody that has been used for treatment of metastatic breast cancer. The antibody is directed against **vascular endothelial growth factor (VEGF)**, a protein that helps tumors form new blood vessels.

Study results for bevacizumab in 2010 did not show a real benefit for women receiving the drug as a part of their treatment. The drug appeared to slow cancer growth for a short time in some women, but it didn't help them live longer and it produced more severe side effects than other drugs.

In late 2010, the FDA announced its plan to remove the breast cancer "indication" for bevacizumab. The drug is still available but cannot be marketed for use in breast cancer. The FDA advised doctors already treating breast cancer patients with the drug to use their medical judgment to decide whether to continue using it or try something else.

Bisphosphonates

Bisphosphonates are drugs that are used to help strengthen and reduce the risk of fractures in bones weakened by metastatic breast cancer. Examples include pamidronate (Aredia) and zoledronic acid (Zometa). They are given intravenously. Bisphosphonates may also help prevent bone thinning (**osteoporosis**) that can result from treatment with aromatase inhibitors or from early menopause caused by chemotherapy. There are a number of medicines, including some oral forms of bisphosphonates, that can treat the loss of bone strength not caused by breast cancer that has spread to the bones.

Bisphosphonates can have side effects, including flu-like symptoms and bone pain. A rare but very distressing side effect of intravenous bisphosphonates is damage in the jawbones (**osteonecrosis** or ONJ). It can be triggered by a tooth extraction (removal) while undergoing treatment with bisphosphonates. ONJ often appears as an open sore in the jaw that will not heal. It can lead to loss of teeth or infections of the jaw bone. Doctors don't know why this happens or how to treat it, other than to stop treatment with bisphosphonates. Maintaining good oral hygiene by flossing, brushing, making sure that dentures fit properly, and having regular dental checkups may help prevent ONJ. Most doctors recommend that patients have a dental checkup and have any tooth or jaw problems treated before they start taking a bisphosphonate.

High-dose Chemotherapy with Stem Cell Transplant

Although it is possible to use very high doses of chemotherapy or radiation to destroy cancer cells, such treatments also kill the blood-making stem cells in the bone marrow. Damage to these cells lowers the blood cell count. A low white blood cell count can lead to severe infections that could be fatal. A low platelet count can make people bleed easily and can also be fatal.

One way to get around these side effects is to remove some of the person's stem cells from either the peripheral (circulating) blood or bone marrow, give the high-dose treatment, and then return the stem cells to the body through a blood transfusion (a process called a **stem cell transplant**). The stem cells are able to find their way back to the bone marrow, where they reestablish themselves and restore the body's ability to make new blood cells.

At one time, it was believed that high-dose chemotherapy with stem cell transplant would be an effective way to treat women with advanced breast cancer. However, several studies have found that women who receive high-dose chemotherapy do not live any longer than women who receive standard chemotherapy without a stem cell transplant. High-dose chemotherapy with stem cell transplant also causes more serious side effects than standard dose chemotherapy. Research is still being done in this area. Although newer studies may show a benefit, it is likely to be small, and toxicity from this type of treatment is very high. At this time, most experts recommend that women with breast cancer should not receive high-dose chemotherapy, except as part of a clinical trial.

Clinical Trials

You probably have had to make many decisions since being told you have cancer. One of the most important decisions you will make is deciding which treatment is best for you. You may have heard about clinical trials being done for your type of cancer. Or maybe someone on your health care team has mentioned a clinical trial to you. Clinical trials are one way to get state-of-the art cancer care. Still, they are not right for everyone.

Here we will give you a brief overview of clinical trials. Talking to your health care team, your family, and your friends can help you make the best treatment choices.

Clinical trials are carefully controlled research studies that are done with patients. These studies test whether a new treatment is safe and how well it works in patients, or they may test new ways to diagnose or prevent a disease. Clinical trials have led to many advances in cancer prevention, diagnosis, and treatment.

Clinical trials are done to get a closer look at promising new treatments or procedures in patients. A clinical trial is undertaken only when there is good reason to believe that the treatment, test, or procedure being studied may be better than the one already being used. Treatments used in clinical trials are often found to have real benefits and may go on to become tomorrow's standard treatment.

Clinical trials can focus on many things:

- new uses of drugs that are already approved by the U.S. Food and Drug Administration (FDA)
- new drugs that have not yet been approved by the FDA
- nondrug treatments (such as radiation therapy)
- medical procedures (such as types of surgery)
- herbs and vitamins
- tools to improve the ways medicines or diagnostic tests are used
- medicines or procedures to relieve symptoms or improve comfort
- combinations of treatments and procedures

Researchers conduct studies of new treatments to try to answer the following questions:

- Is the treatment helpful?
- What's the best way to give it?
- Does it work better than other treatments already available?
- What side effects does the treatment cause?
- Are there more or fewer side effects than the standard treatment used now?
- Do the benefits outweigh the side effects?
- In which patients is the treatment most likely to be helpful?

Clinical trials are usually conducted in distinct phases. Each phase is designed to answer certain questions. Knowing the phase of the clinical trial is important because it can give you some idea about how much is known about the treatment being studied. There are pros and cons to taking part in each phase of a clinical trial.

Phase 0 clinical trials

Even though phase 0 studies are done in humans, this type of study is different from the other phases of clinical trials. However, some cancer patients probably will be asked to take part in these kinds of studies in the future.

Phase 0 studies are exploratory studies that often use only a few small doses of a new drug in each patient. The studies are done to find out whether the drug reaches the tumor, how the drug acts in the human body, and how cancer cells respond to the drug. The patients in these studies must have extra biopsies, scans, and blood tests. The biggest difference between phase 0 and later phases of clinical trials is that there is no chance of a direct benefit to the patient in a phase 0 trial. Because drug doses are low, there is also less risk to the patient in phase 0 studies compared with phase I studies.

Phase 0 studies help researchers learn which drugs do act as expected. If there are problems with the way the drug is absorbed or acts in the body, this should become clear very quickly in a phase 0 trial.

Phase 0 studies are not yet being used widely, and there are some drugs for which they would not be helpful. The studies are very small, mostly with fewer than 20 people. They are not a required part of testing a new drug but are part of an effort to speed up and streamline the process.

Phase I clinical trials

The purpose of a phase I study is to find the safest way to give a new treatment to patients. The cancer care team closely watches patients for any harmful side effects.

For phase I studies, the drug has already been tested in laboratory and animal studies, but the side effects in patients are not fully known. Doctors start by giving very low doses of the drug to the first patients and increase the doses for later groups of patients until side effects appear or the desired effect is seen. Doctors are hoping to help the study patients, but the main purpose of a phase I trial is to test the safety of the drug.

Phase I clinical trials are often done in small groups of people with different cancers that have not responded to standard treatment, or that keep coming back (recurring) after treatment. If a drug is found to be reasonably safe in phase I studies, it can be tested in a phase II clinical trial.

Phase II clinical trials

These studies are designed to see whether the drug is effective. Patients are given the most appropriate (safest) dose as determined from phase I studies. They are closely watched for an effect on the cancer. The cancer care team also looks for side effects. Phase II trials are often done in larger groups of patients with a specific cancer type that has not responded to standard treatment. If a drug is found to be effective in phase II studies, it can be tested in a phase III clinical trial.

Phase III clinical trials

Phase III studies involve large numbers of patients—most often those patients who have just received a diagnosis for a specific type of cancer. Phase III clinical trials may enroll thousands of patients. Often, these studies are **randomized**, which means that patients are randomly put in 1 of 2 (or more) groups. One group (called the **control group**) gets the standard, most accepted treatment. The other group(s) gets the new treatment(s) being studied. All patients in phase III studies are closely watched. The study will be stopped early if many patients have side effects from the new treatment that are too severe or if one group has much better results than the others. Phase III clinical trials are needed before the FDA will approve a treatment for use by the general public.

Phase IV clinical trials

Once a drug has been approved by the FDA and is available for all patients, it is still studied in other clinical trials (sometimes referred to as phase IV studies). This way, more can be learned about short-term and long-term side effects and safety as the drug is used in larger numbers of patients with many types of diseases. Doctors can also learn more about how well the drug works and whether it might be helpful when used in other ways (such as in combination with other treatments).

What it is like to be in a clinical trial

If you participate in a clinical trial, you will have a team of cancer care experts taking care of you and watching your progress very carefully. Depending on the phase of the clinical trial, you may receive more attention (such as having more doctor visits and laboratory tests) than you would if you were treated outside of a clinical trial. Clinical trials are designed to pay close attention to you. However, there are some risks. No one involved in the study knows in advance whether the treatment will work or exactly what side effects will occur. That outcome is what the study is designed to find out. While most side effects go away in time, some may be long-lasting or even life-threatening. Keep in mind, though, that even standard treatments have side effects.

Deciding to enter a clinical trial

If you would like to take part in a clinical trial, you should begin by asking your doctor if your clinic or hospital conducts clinical trials. There are requirements you must meet to take part in any clinical trial. But whether or not you enter (enroll in) a clinical trial is completely up to you. The doctors and nurses conducting the study will explain the study to you in detail. They will go over the possible risks and benefits and give you a form (**informed consent**) to read and sign. The form says that you understand the clinical trial and want to take part in it. Even after you read and sign the form and after the clinical trial begins, you are free to leave the study at any time, for any reason. Taking part in a clinical trial does not keep you from getting any other medical care you may need.

To find out more about clinical trials, talk to your cancer care team. Here are some questions you might ask:

- Is there a clinical trial that I should take part in?
- What is the purpose of the study?
- How might this study be of benefit to me?
- What is likely to happen in my case with, or without, this new treatment?
- What kinds of tests and treatments does the study involve?
- What does this treatment do? Has it been used before?
- Will I know which treatment I receive?
- What are my other choices and their pros and cons?
- How could the study affect my daily life?
- What side effects can I expect from the study? Can the side effects be controlled?
- Will I have to stay in the hospital? If so, how often and for how long?
- Will the study cost me anything? Will any of the treatment be free?
- If I am harmed as a result of the research, what treatment would I be entitled to?
- What type of long-term follow-up care is part of the study?
- Has the treatment been used to treat other types of cancer?

How can I find out more about clinical trials that might be right for me?

The American Cancer Society offers a clinical trials matching service for use by patients, their family, or friends. You can reach this service at **800-303-5691** or on the Web at **http://clinicaltrials .cancer.org**.

Based on the information you give about your cancer type, stage, and previous treatments, this service can put together a list of clinical trials that match your medical needs. The service will also ask where you live and whether you are willing to travel so that it can look for a treatment center that you can get to. You can also get a list of current clinical trials by calling the National Cancer Institute's Cancer Information Service toll-free at **800-4-CANCER (800-422-6237)** or by visiting the NCI clinical trials Web site at **www.cancer .gov/clinicaltrials**.

For even more information on clinical trials, see the American Cancer Society document *Clinical Trials: What You Need to Know,* available on the Web at **cancer.org**. You may also request this document by calling our toll-free number, **800-227-2345**.

Complementary and Alternative Treatments

When you have cancer, you are likely to hear about ways to treat your cancer or relieve symptoms that are different from mainstream (standard) medical treatment. These treatments can include vitamins, herbs, and special diets, or acupuncture and massage—among many others. You may have a lot of questions about these treatments. Talk to your doctor about any treatment you are considering. Here are some questions to ask:

- How do I know if the treatment is safe?
- How do I know if it works?
- Should I try one or more of these treatments?
- Will these treatments cause a problem with my standard medical treatment?
- What is the difference between complementary and alternative treatments?
- Where can I find out more about these treatments?

The terms can be confusing

Not everyone uses these terms the same way, so it can be confusing. The American Cancer Society uses **complementary therapy** to refer to medicines or treatments that are used *along with* your regular medical care. **Alternative therapy** is a treatment used *instead of* standard medical treatment.

Complementary treatments

Complementary treatment methods, for the most part, are not presented as cures for cancer. Most often they are used to help you feel better. Some methods that can be used in a complementary way are meditation to reduce stress, acupuncture to relieve pain, or peppermint tea to relieve nausea. There are many others. Some of these methods are known to help and could add to your comfort and well being, while others have not been tested.

Some have been proven not to be helpful. A few have even been found harmful. There are many complementary methods that you can safely use right along with your medical treatment to help relieve symptoms or side effects, to ease pain, and to help you enjoy life more. For example, some people find methods such as aromatherapy, massage therapy, meditation, or yoga to be useful.

Alternative treatments

Alternative treatments are those methods that are used instead of standard medical care. These treatments have not been proven to be safe and effective in clinical trials. Some of these treatments may even be dangerous or have life-threatening side effects. The biggest danger in most cases is that you may lose the chance to benefit from standard treatment. Delays or interruptions in your standard medical treatment may give the cancer more time to grow.

Deciding what to do

It is easy to see why people with cancer may consider alternative treatments. You want to do all you can to fight the cancer. Sometimes mainstream treatments such as chemotherapy can be hard to take, or they may no longer be working. Sometimes people suggest that their treatment can cure your cancer without having serious side effects, and it's normal to want to believe them. But the truth is that most nonstandard treatments have not been tested and proven to be effective for treating cancer.

As you consider your options, here are 3 important steps you can take:

- Talk to your doctor or nurse about any treatment you are thinking about using.
- Check the list of "red flags," below.
- Contact the American Cancer Society at **800-227-2345** to learn more about complementary and alternative treatments in general and to learn more about the specific treatments you are considering.

Red flags

You can use the questions below to spot treatments or methods to avoid. A "yes" answer to any one of these questions should raise a red flag.

- Does the treatment promise a cure?
- Are you told not to use standard medical treatment?
- Is the treatment or drug a "secret" that only certain people can give?
- Does the treatment require you to travel to another country?
- Do the promoters attack the medical or scientific community?

The decision is yours

Decisions about how to treat or manage your cancer are always yours to make. If you are thinking about using a complementary or alternative method, be sure to learn about it and talk with your doctor about it. With reliable information and the support of your health care team, you may be able to safely use methods that can help you while avoiding those that could be harmful.

Treatment of Breast Cancer According to Stage

Treatment of Noninvasive (Stage 0) Breast Cancer

The 2 types of noninvasive breast cancers, lobular carcinoma in situ (LCIS) and ductal carcinoma in situ (DCIS), are treated very differently.

Lobular carcinoma in situ

No immediate or active treatment is recommended for most women with lobular carcinoma in situ (LCIS), as this condition is not considered a true cancer. However, having LCIS increases the risk that invasive cancer will develop later, so close follow-up is very important. This follow-up usually includes yearly mammograms and clinical breast examinations. Women with LCIS may also want to talk with their doctors about the benefits and limits of being screened yearly with magnetic resonance imaging (MRI) in addition to mammograms. Close monitoring of both breasts is important because women with LCIS in one breast have the same increased risk for cancer to develop in either breast.

Women with LCIS may also want to consider taking tamoxifen or raloxifene to reduce their risk of breast cancer or may consider taking part in a clinical trial for breast cancer prevention. For more information on drugs to reduce breast cancer risk, contact your American Cancer Society at **800-227-2345** and ask for the document *Medicines to Reduce Breast Cancer Risk,* or visit our Web site, **cancer.org**.

Women with LCIS should also discuss other possible prevention strategies (such as reaching an optimal body weight or starting an exercise program) with their doctors. Some women with LCIS choose to have a bilateral simple mastectomy (removal of both breasts but not axillary lymph nodes), especially if they have other risk factors, such as a strong family history of breast cancer.

Ductal carcinoma in situ

In most cases, a woman with ductal carcinoma in situ (DCIS) can choose between breast-conserving therapy (a lumpectomy, usually followed by radiation therapy) and simple mastectomy. Lymph node removal (axillary dissection) is usually not needed. A lumpectomy without radiation therapy is an option only for women in whom a small area of low-grade DCIS was removed with large enough cancer-free surgical margins. Most women who have a lumpectomy, however, will require radiation therapy.

Mastectomy may be necessary if the area of DCIS is very large, if there are several areas of DCIS within the breast, or if the DCIS cannot be completely removed by lumpectomy (if the lumpectomy specimen and reexcision specimens have cancer cells in the surgical margins).

If the DCIS is estrogen receptor–positive, treatment with tamoxifen for 5 years after surgery can lower the risk that another DCIS or invasive cancer will develop in either breast. Women should discuss the advantages and disadvantages of this option with their doctors.

Treatment of Invasive Breast Cancer by Stage

Breast-conserving surgery is sometimes appropriate for early-stage invasive breast cancer if the tumor is small enough, although mastectomy is also an option. If the tumor is too large, a mastectomy will be needed unless neoadjuvant chemotherapy can shrink the tumor enough to allow breast-conserving surgery. In either case, the lymph nodes will need to be checked and removed if they contain cancer. Radiation will be needed for almost all women who have breast-conserving surgery and for some who have mastectomies. Adjuvant systemic therapy after surgery is typically recommended if the tumor is larger than 1 cm (about ½ inch) and for some tumors that are smaller than 1 cm.

Stage I

Stage I cancers are still relatively small and have not spread to the lymph nodes or elsewhere.

Local therapy: Stage I cancers can be treated with breast-conserving surgery (lumpectomy or partial mastectomy) or modified radical mastectomy. The lymph nodes will also need to be evaluated with a sentinel lymph node biopsy or axillary lymph node dissection. Breast reconstruction can be done at the same time as surgery or later.

Radiation therapy is usually given after breast-conserving surgery. Women who may consider breast-conserving surgery *without* radiation therapy typically have all of the following characteristics:

- They are age 70 or older.
- Their tumor was 2 cm or smaller and has been completely removed.
- Their tumor contains hormone receptors and they have received hormone therapy.
- There is no lymph node involvement.

Although some women who do not meet these criteria may be tempted to avoid radiation, studies have shown that not undergoing radiation therapy increases the chances of a recurrence.

Adjuvant systemic therapy: Most doctors will discuss the advantages and disadvantages of adjuvant hormone therapy (either tamoxifen or an aromatase inhibitor) with all women who have a hormone receptor–positive breast cancer, no matter how small the tumor. Women with tumors larger than 0.5 cm (about ¼ inch) may be more likely to benefit from adjuvant hormone therapy.

Adjuvant chemotherapy is not usually offered if the tumor is smaller than 1 cm (about ½ inch). Some doctors may suggest adjuvant chemotherapy if a tumor smaller than 1 cm has any unfavorable features (for example, high grade, hormone receptor–negative, HER2-positive, or a high score on one of the gene pattern tests). Adjuvant chemotherapy is usually recommended for larger tumors.

For HER2-positive cancers, adjuvant trastuzumab (Herceptin) is usually recommended as well.

Stage II

Stage II cancers are larger and/or have spread to a few nearby lymph nodes.

Local therapy: Surgery and radiation therapy options for stage II cancers are similar to those for stage I tumors. For stage II cancers, however, radiation therapy may be considered after mastectomy if the tumor is larger than 5 cm or if the cancer cells are found in several lymph nodes.

Adjuvant systemic therapy: Adjuvant systemic therapy is recommended for women with stage II breast cancer. It may involve hormone therapy, chemotherapy, trastuzumab, or some combination of these therapies, depending on the woman's age, whether the cancer is ER– or PR–positive, and the cancer's HER2/neu status.

Neoadjuvant therapy: An option for some women who would like to have breast-conserving therapy for tumors larger than 2 cm (about $\frac{4}{5}$ inch in width) is to have neoadjuvant (presurgical) chemotherapy, hormone therapy, and/or trastuzumab to shrink the tumor. If the neoadjuvant treatment shrinks the tumor enough, the woman may be able to have breast-conserving surgery (such as a lumpectomy) followed by radiation therapy and/or hormone therapy (if the tumor is hormone receptor–positive). Further chemotherapy may also be considered.

If the neoadjuvant therapy does not cause the tumor to shrink enough for breast-conserving surgery to be an option, a mastectomy may be required. This mastectomy may be followed by a different type of chemotherapy.

If the tumor is large (more than 2 inches in size) or if there is lymph node involvement, radiation therapy may be needed. Radiation is usually given after surgery. Hormone therapy may be given if the tumor is hormone receptor–positive. Hormone therapy can be given both before and after surgery. A woman's chance for surviving breast cancer does not appear to be affected by whether she undergoes chemotherapy before or after breast surgery.

Stage III

Local treatment for some stage IIIA breast cancers is largely the same as treatment for stage II breast cancers. The cancer may be removed by breast-conserving surgery (such as a lumpectomy) with follow-up radiation therapy, or it may be removed by modified radical mastectomy (with or without breast reconstruction). Sentinel lymph node biopsy or axillary lymph node dissection is also done. Radiation therapy may be used after mastectomy if the tumor is larger than 5 cm or if the cancer has spread to several lymph nodes. Neoadjuvant therapy may be an option for women who would like to have breast-conserving surgery. Surgery is usually followed by adjuvant chemotherapy, hormone therapy, and/or trastuzumab.

Stage III cancers are often treated with neoadjuvant chemotherapy (chemotherapy before surgery). Then, a mastectomy is done, usually with removal of the axillary lymph nodes (an axillary lymph node dissection). Reconstruction may be done as well. Breast-conserving surgery may be an option for some women. Surgery is followed by radiation therapy, even if the woman has had a mastectomy. Adjuvant chemotherapy may also be given, and adjuvant hormone therapy is offered to all women with hormone receptor–positive breast cancers.

Adjuvant therapy for stages I to III breast cancer

Adjuvant drug therapy may be recommended for women with stage I, II, or III breast cancer, based on the tumor's size, whether it has spread to lymph nodes, and other features. If adjuvant therapy is recommended, this therapy might include chemotherapy, trastuzumab (Herceptin), hormone therapy, or some combination of these.

Hormone therapy: Hormone therapy is not likely to be effective for women with hormone receptor–negative tumors. Hormone therapy is likely to be offered to all women with hormone receptor–positive invasive breast cancer, regardless of the size of the tumor or the number of lymph nodes involved.

Premenopausal women who have hormone receptor–positive tumors can be treated with tamoxifen, which blocks the effects of the estrogen made by the ovaries. Some doctors also give a luteinizing hormone-releasing hormone (LHRH) analog, which makes the ovaries temporarily stop functioning. Another option, though permanent, is surgical removal of the ovaries (oophorectomy). If the woman becomes postmenopausal within 5 years of starting tamoxifen (either naturally or because her ovaries are removed), she may be switched from tamoxifen to an aromatase inhibitor.

Aromatase inhibitors will only benefit postmenopausal women. Sometimes a woman's menstrual periods will stop after chemotherapy or while the woman is taking tamoxifen. But this does not necessarily mean the woman is truly postmenopausal. Menopausal status can be determined by blood tests for certain hormones.

Women no longer having periods or who are known to be in menopause and who have hormone receptor–positive tumors will generally receive adjuvant hormone therapy—either with an aromatase inhibitor (typically for 5 years) or with tamoxifen for a few years, followed by an aromatase inhibitor for a few more. Women who cannot take aromatase inhibitors may instead take tamoxifen for 5 years.

There are still many unanswered questions about the best way to use aromatase inhibitors and tamoxifen. For example, it is unclear whether starting adjuvant therapy with an aromatase inhibitor is better than giving tamoxifen for some length of time and then switching to an aromatase inhibitor. Nor has the optimal length of treatment with aromatase inhibitors been determined. Studies now under way should help answer these questions. You may want to discuss these newer treatments with your doctor.

As a general rule, hormone therapy is given after any chemotherapy treatments have been completed.

Chemotherapy: Chemotherapy is usually recommended for all women with invasive breast cancer that is hormone receptor–negative. Women who have hormone receptor–positive tumors may get additional benefit from undergoing chemotherapy with hormone therapy, based on the stage and characteristics of their cancer.

Adjuvant chemotherapy can decrease the risk of recurrence, but it does not remove all risk. Before deciding whether adjuvant chemotherapy is right for you, it is important to understand your personal risk for cancer recurrence and the extent to which adjuvant therapy will decrease that risk.

The specific drug regimens and the length of treatment are often determined by the stage and grade of the cancer. Typical chemotherapy regimens are listed in the chemotherapy section on pages 143–145. The length of these regimens usually ranges from 4 to 6 months. In some cases, dose-dense chemotherapy may be used (see pages 145–146 for more information on dose-dense chemotherapy).

Trastuzumab: For women with HER2-positive cancers, trastuzumab is usually administered along with chemotherapy. A common chemotherapy regimen is a combination of doxorubicin and cyclophosphamide for approximately 3 months, followed by paclitaxel for approximately 3 months. Trastuzumab would be given with the chemotherapy and continue for approximately 1 year.

A concern among doctors is that taking trastuzumab so soon after doxorubicin can lead to heart problems, so heart function is monitored closely during treatment by using echocardiograms or other cardiac tests. To lessen possible damage to the heart, doctors are also looking for effective chemotherapy combinations that do not contain doxorubicin. One such regimen is called "TCH."

With TCH, the person receives a combination of docetaxel and carboplatin every 3 weeks along with weekly trastuzumab. There are typically 6 cycles of the chemotherapy drugs. The 6-cycle treatment period is followed by an additional year of trastuzumab given every 3 weeks.

Making decisions about adjuvant therapy: Some doctors may use newer gene pattern tests to help decide whether adjuvant chemotherapy will be beneficial for women with stage I or II breast cancer. Examples of such tests include Oncotype DX and MammaPrint, which are described in more detail in the section "How Is Breast Cancer Diagnosed?" on pages 89–90. Gene pattern tests require a sample of your breast cancer tissue. The function of genes within the cancer is studied so that the doctor can better predict the risk for cancer recurrence after treatment. However, gene pattern tests will not provide enough information for your doctor to know definitively which hormone therapy or chemotherapy is best for you. Clinical trials are under way to evaluate the usefulness of gene pattern tests in certain situations—for example, in women with small tumors where there is no lymph node involvement.

For help in deciding whether adjuvant therapy is right for you, visit the Mayo Clinic Web site at www.mayoclinic.com and type "adjuvant therapy for breast cancer" into the search box. This Web site is an excellent source of information on the possible benefits and limits of adjuvant therapy. Other online guides, such as www.adjuvant online.com, are designed to be used by health care professionals. This Web site provides information about risk of cancer recurrence within 10 years and what benefits one might expect from hormone therapy and/or chemotherapy. You may want to ask your doctor his or her opinion of this site.

Stage IV

Stage IV cancers have spread beyond the breast and lymph nodes to other parts of the body. Although surgery and/or radiation may be useful in some situations, they are very unlikely to cure these cancers. Therefore, systemic therapy is the main treatment. Depending on many factors, this treatment may include hormone therapy, chemotherapy, targeted therapies such as trastuzumab or bevacizumab, or some combination of these treatments.

Trastuzumab may extend life for women with stage IV HER2-positive cancer if it is given with the first chemotherapy dose. It is not known whether giving trastuzumab at the same time as hormone therapy has this same benefit or for how long a woman should remain on trastuzumab.

Bevacizumab, a drug that blocks new tumor blood vessel growth, was previously used for treatment of advanced breast cancer; however, the FDA has recommended it not be used for this indication. See the section "Targeted Therapy" on page 156 for more information on this drug.

All systemic therapies—hormone therapy, chemotherapy, and the newer targeted therapies— have potential side effects. Your doctor will explain the benefits and risks of these treatments before prescribing them.

Radiation therapy and/or surgery may also be used in certain situations, such as to treat metastases in certain areas, to prevent bone fractures or blockage in the liver, or to provide relief of pain or other symptoms. If your doctor recommends local treatment, it is important that you understand its goal—whether it is to try to cure the cancer or to prevent or treat symptoms. In some cases, regional chemotherapy (where drugs are delivered directly into a certain area, such as into the fluid around the brain) may be useful as well.

Treatment to relieve symptoms depends on where the cancer has spread. For example, pain from bone metastases may be treated with external beam radiation therapy and/or bisphosphonates such as pamidronate or zoledronic acid. Most doctors recommend bisphosphonates, along with calcium and vitamin D, for all patients with bone metastases. For more information about treatment of bone metastases, contact your American Cancer Society at **800-227-2345** and request the document *Bone Metastasis,* or visit our Web site, **cancer.org**.

Advanced cancer that progresses during treatment: Although treatment for advanced breast cancer can shrink or slow the growth of the cancer (often for many years), it may stop working at some point. Further treatment then depends on several factors, including previous treatments, the cancer's location, and the woman's age, general health, and desire to continue treatment.

For hormone receptor–positive cancers that were being treated with hormone therapy, switching to another type of hormone therapy is sometimes helpful. If not, chemotherapy is usually the next step. For cancers that are no longer responding to one chemotherapy regimen, trying another regimen may be helpful. There are many different drugs and combinations that can be used to treat breast cancer. However, each time a cancer progresses during treatment, it becomes less likely that further treatment will have an effect.

HER2-positive cancers that no longer respond to trastuzumab may respond to lapatinib, another drug that attacks the HER2 protein. This drug is usually given with the chemotherapy drug capecitabine. Both of these drugs are taken as pills.

Current treatments are very unlikely to cure advanced breast cancer. Women in otherwise good health are encouraged to think about taking part in clinical trials of other promising treatments.

Recurrent breast cancer

When cancer comes back after treatment, it is said to be recurrent. Recurrence can be local (in the same breast or near the mastectomy scar) or in a distant area. Cancer that is found in the opposite breast is not a recurrence—it is a new cancer that requires its own distinct treatment.

Local recurrence: Treatment of women whose breast cancer has recurred locally depends on their initial treatment. If the woman had breast-conserving therapy, local recurrence in the breast is usually treated with mastectomy. If the initial treatment was mastectomy, a recurrence near the mastectomy site will be treated by removing the tumor whenever possible. If the woman did not receive radiation therapy after the first surgery, she will undergo radiation. (Radiation cannot be given to the same area twice.) In either case, hormone therapy, trastuzumab, chemotherapy, or some combination of these may be used after surgery and/or radiation therapy.

Distant recurrence: In general, women who have a recurrence involving organs such as the bones, lungs, or brain are treated the same way as women who are found to have stage IV breast cancer that has spread to these organs when it is diagnosed (see treatment for stage IV, page 183). The only difference is that treatment may be affected by any previous treatments the woman has had.

For more information on how to manage and cope with a cancer recurrence, contact your American Cancer Society at **800-227-2345** to request the document *When Your Cancer Comes Back: Cancer Recurrence,* or visit our Web site, **cancer.org**.

Treatment of Breast Cancer During Pregnancy

Breast cancer is diagnosed in about 1 of 3,000 pregnant women. In general, treatment recommendations depend upon the stage of pregnancy at the time of diagnosis. Radiation therapy during pregnancy is known to increase the risk of birth defects, so it is not recommended for pregnant women with breast cancer. For this reason, breast-conserving therapy (lumpectomy and radiation therapy) is an option only if treatment can be delayed until the baby can be delivered safely. However, breast biopsy procedures and even modified radical mastectomy are safe for the mother and fetus.

For many years, it was assumed that chemotherapy was dangerous to the fetus. However, several recent studies have found that using certain chemotherapy drugs during the second and third trimesters (the fourth to ninth months of pregnancy) does not increase the risk of birth defects. Because of concern about the potential damage to the fetus, the safety of chemotherapy during the first trimester (the first 3 months of pregnancy) has not been studied.

Hormone therapy may affect the fetus and should not be started until after the woman has given birth. Many chemotherapy and hormone therapy drugs can enter breast milk and could be passed on to the baby, so breastfeeding is not usually recommended during chemotherapy or hormone therapy. For more information on breast cancer and pregnancy, contact your American Cancer Society at **800-227-2345** and request the document *Pregnancy and Breast Cancer,* or visit our Web site, **cancer.org**.

More Treatment Information

For more details on treatment options—including some that may not be addressed in this book—the

National Cancer Institute (NCI) and the National Comprehensive Cancer Network (NCCN) are good sources of information. The NCI provides treatment guidelines via its telephone information center (800-4-CANCER) and its Web site (www.cancer.gov). Detailed guidelines intended for use by cancer care professionals are also available on www.cancer.gov. The NCCN, made up of experts from many of the nation's leading cancer centers, develops cancer treatment guidelines for doctors to use when treating patients. Those are available on the NCCN Web site (www.nccn.org).

Breast Reconstruction

If you are thinking about having reconstructive surgery, it is a good idea to talk about it with your surgeon and plastic surgeon before your mastectomy. This lets the surgical teams plan the treatment that is best for you, even if you want to wait and have reconstructive surgery later.

The choice to have breast reconstruction is yours. No one source of information can give you all the answers. Talk about the benefits and risks of reconstruction with your doctors, and give yourself plenty of time to make a decision. You should decide to have breast reconstruction only after you are fully informed.

Immediate or Delayed Breast Reconstruction

Immediate breast reconstruction is done at the same time as the mastectomy. An advantage to this option is that the chest tissues are not damaged by scarring, which can mean the final result will look better. Immediate reconstruction means less surgery. Immediate reconstruction is more likely to be an option if the woman does not need to have radiation therapy after surgery. After the first surgery, there still may be a number of steps that are needed to complete the immediate reconstruction process. If you are planning to have immediate reconstruction, ask what will need to be done afterward and how long it will take.

Delayed breast reconstruction means that the rebuilding is started later. This may be a better choice for women who need radiation to the chest area after the mastectomy. Radiation therapy given after breast reconstruction surgery can cause problems.

Types of Breast Reconstruction

Breast reconstruction can be done by using a **breast implant**, tissue taken from somewhere else on your body, or a combination of the two.

Implant procedures

The most common type of implant is a silicone shell filled with sterile saline (salt water). Silicone gel–filled implants are another option for breast reconstruction. There has been a decline in the use of silicone implants because of concerns that silicone leakage might cause immune system diseases. However, most recent studies show that silicone implants do not increase the risk of immune system problems. Clinical trials are currently under way to study alternative breast implants that have different shells and are filled with different materials.

One-stage immediate breast reconstruction may be done at the same time as mastectomy. After the general surgeon removes the breast tissue, a plastic surgeon places the breast implant where the breast tissue was removed.

Two-stage reconstruction (also called two-stage delayed reconstruction or delayed-immediate reconstruction) is done if your skin and chest wall tissues are tight and flat. An implanted **tissue expander**, which is like a balloon, is put under the skin and chest muscle. Over the course of 4 to 6 months, the surgeon will inject a saline solution through a tiny valve under the skin to fill the expander. After the skin over the breast area has stretched adequately, a second surgery will be done to remove the expander and put in the implant. In some cases, the expander is left in place as the final implant.

The two-stage reconstruction allows more flexibility. If surgical biopsies show that radiation is needed, the next steps of reconstruction can be delayed until radiation treatment is complete.

There are some important factors for you to keep in mind if you are thinking about having implants:

- Implants may not last a lifetime. You may need more surgery to replace them later.
- You can have problems with breast implants. They can rupture or cause infection or pain.
- Scar tissue may form around the implant or you may not like the way the implant looks.

- Breast reconstruction restores the shape, but not feeling, in the breast. With time, the skin on the reconstructed breast can become more sensitive, but it will not feel the same as it did before your mastectomy.

The surgeon may recommend surgery to reshape the remaining breast to match the reconstructed breast. This could include reducing or enlarging the size of the breast or even surgically lifting the breast.

Tissue flap procedures

Tissue flap reconstruction uses tissue from your abdomen, back, thighs, or buttocks to rebuild the breast. The 2 most common types of tissue flap surgeries are the transverse rectus abdominis muscle flap, or TRAM flap, which uses tissue from the abdominal area, and the latissimus dorsi flap, or LAT flap, which uses tissue from the upper back.

These operations leave 2 surgical sites and scars—one where the tissue was taken and one on the reconstructed breast. The scars fade over time, but they never go away completely. There can be problems at the donor site, such as abdominal hernias or muscle damage or weakness. There may be differences in the size and shape of the breasts. Because healthy blood vessels are needed for the supply blood to the transplanted tissue, flap procedures are not usually offered to women with diabetes, connective tissue disease, vascular disease, or to women who smoke.

In general, breast reconstruction done by flap procedure will create a breast that behaves more like the rest of your body tissue. For example, the breast may enlarge or shrink if you gain or lose weight. There is also no worry about replacement or rupture.

Transverse rectus abdominis muscle flap: The transverse rectus abdominis muscle flap, or **TRAM flap**, procedure uses tissue and muscle from the lower abdominal wall. Tissue from this area alone is often enough to form the breast, and an implant may not be needed. The skin, fat, blood vessels, and at least one abdominal muscle are

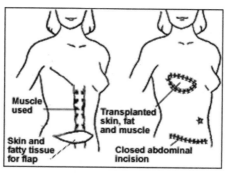

TRAM Flap Incisions

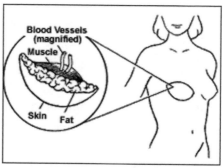

Tissue Used to Rebuild Breast Shape

moved from the abdomen to the chest. The TRAM flap procedure can cause a decrease in abdominal strength and may not be possible in women who have had abdominal tissue removed in previous surgeries. The procedure also results in a tightening of the lower abdomen, or a "tummy tuck."

There are 2 types of TRAM flaps:

- In a **pedicle flap,** the tissue remains attached to its original blood supply and is tunneled under the skin to the breast area.

- In a **free flap**, the surgeon cuts the skin, fat, blood vessels, and muscle free from their original location and then attaches them to blood vessels in the chest. This requires the use of microsurgery to connect the tiny vessels and takes longer than a pedicle flap. The free flap procedure is not done as often as the pedicle flap, but some doctors think that it results in a more natural shape.

Latissimus dorsi flap: The latissimus dorsi flap, or **LAT flap**, moves muscle and skin from your upper back to the chest area. The flap is made up of skin, fat, muscle, and blood vessels. The tissue is tunneled under the skin to the front of the chest. This creates a pocket for an implant, which can be used to add fullness to the reconstructed breast. Some women may have weakness in their back, shoulder, or arm after this surgery, but this is not common.

Deep inferior epigastric artery perforator flap: A newer type of flap procedure, the deep

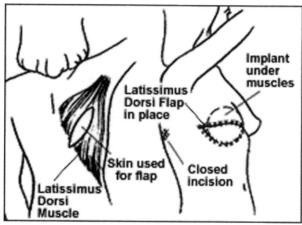

Latissimus Dorsi Flap

inferior epigastric artery perforator flap, or **DIEP flap**, uses fat and skin from the abdominal area (as in the TRAM flap) but it does not use the abdominal muscle. The DIEP flap procedure uses a free flap, meaning that the tissue is completely cut free from the abdomen and moved to the chest area. Microsurgery is required to connect the tiny vessels. The procedure takes longer than the TRAM pedicle flap. The DIEP flap procedure results in a tightening of the lower abdomen, or a "tummy tuck."

Gluteal free flap: The gluteal free flap or superior gluteal artery perforator (SGAP) flap is a newer type of surgery that uses tissue from the buttocks, including the gluteal muscle, to create the breast shape. The SGAP flap is an option for women who cannot or do not wish to use the abdominal site because of thinness, incisions, or other reasons.

The method is much like the TRAM free flap. The skin, fat, blood vessels, and muscle are cut out of the buttocks and moved to the chest area. Microsurgery is used to connect the tiny vessels.

New methods of tissue support

All of the reconstructive surgeries just discussed move sections of tissue to new places or place fairly heavy implants in the body, and the body tissue needs support as it heals. Doctors use synthetic mesh and other methods for this support. More recently, doctors are trying a new product called AlloDerm, which is made of donated human skin. It is regulated by the U.S. Food and Drug Administration (FDA) as a human tissue used for transplant. It is acellular, meaning it has had the human cells removed that can carry diseases or lead to rejection by the body. It is used to extend and support natural tissues and help them grow and heal. In breast reconstruction, it may be used with expanders and implants. It has also been used in nipple reconstruction. AlloDerm is a fairly new product; studies that look at outcomes are still in progress but have been promising. AlloDerm is not used by every plastic surgeon, but is becoming more widely available.

Nipple and Areola Reconstruction

You can decide whether you want to have your nipple and areola reconstructed. Nipple and areola reconstructions are optional and are usually the final phase of breast reconstruction. This is a separate surgery and is done to make the reconstructed breast look more like the original breast. It can be done as an outpatient procedure under local anesthesia. It is usually done about 3 to 4 months after surgery, once the new breast has had time to heal.

Ideally, the position, size, shape, texture, color, and projection of the new nipple will match the natural one. Tissue used to rebuild the nipple and areola also is taken from your body, such as from the newly created breast, opposite nipple, ear, eyelid, groin, upper inner thigh, or buttocks. A tattoo may be used to match the color of the nipple of the other breast and to create the areola.

Nipple-sparing procedures

In a newer procedure called nipple-sparing mastectomy, the nipple and areola are left in place while the breast tissue under them is removed. For more information about this procedure, see pages 122–123.

Choosing Your Plastic Surgeon

Once you decide to have breast reconstruction, you will need to find a board-certified plastic surgeon with experience in breast reconstruction. Your breast surgeon can suggest doctors for you. To find out whether a surgeon is board certified, contact the American Society of Plastic Surgeons (ASPS). This organization has a Plastic Surgery Information Service that provides a list of ASPS members in a caller's area who are certified by the American Board of Plastic Surgery. See the Resources section on page 247 for contact information.

Questions to ask your plastic surgeon

It is very important that you get all of your questions answered by your plastic surgeon before having breast reconstruction. If you don't understand something, ask your surgeon about it. Here is a list of questions to get you started. Write down other questions as you think of them. You may want to record your talks with your surgeon or take notes. Some people bring a friend or family member with them to the doctor to help remember what was said. The answers to these questions may help you make your decisions.

- Can I have breast reconstruction?
- When can I have reconstruction done?
- What types of reconstruction could I have?
- What is the average cost of each type? Will my insurance cover them?
- What type of reconstruction do you think would be best for me? Why?
- How many of these procedures have you (plastic surgeon) done?
- What results can I expect?
- Will the reconstructed breast match my other breast?
- How will my reconstructed breast feel to the touch?
- Will I have any feeling in my reconstructed breast?
- What possible problems should I know about?
- How much discomfort or pain will I feel?

- How long will I be in the hospital?
- Will I need blood transfusions? If so, can I donate my own blood?
- How long will it take for me to recover?
- What will I need to do at home to care for my incisions (surgical wounds)?
- Will I have a drain (tube that lets fluid out) when I go home?
- How much help will I need at home to take care of my drain and wound?
- When can I start my exercises?
- How much activity can I do at home?
- When will I be able to go back to normal activity such as driving and working?
- Can I talk with other women who have had the same surgery?
- Will reconstruction interfere with chemotherapy?
- Will reconstruction interfere with radiation therapy?
- How long will the implant last?
- What kinds of changes to the breast can I expect over time?
- How will aging affect the reconstructed breast?
- What happens if I gain or lose weight?
- Are there any new reconstruction options that I should know about?

It is common to get a second opinion before having any surgery. Breast reconstruction and even mastectomy are not emergencies. It is more important for you to make the right decisions based on the correct information than to act quickly before you know all your options.

Before Surgery

Planning your surgery

You can start talking about reconstruction as soon as you know you have breast cancer. You will want your breast surgeon and your plastic surgeon to work together to come up with the best possible plan for reconstruction. After reviewing your medical history and overall health, your surgeon will explain which reconstructive options are best for you based on your age, health, body type, lifestyle, and goals. Talk with your surgeon openly about what you expect. Your surgeon should be frank with you when explaining the risks and benefits of each option.

Breast reconstruction after a mastectomy can make you feel better about how you look and renew your self-confidence. But keep in mind that the reconstructed breast will not be a perfect match or substitute for your natural breast. If tissue from your abdomen, back, or buttocks is used, those areas will look different after surgery. Talk with your surgeon about scars and changes in shape or contour. Ask where they will be and how they will look and feel after they heal.

Health insurance policies often cover most or all of the cost of reconstruction after a mastectomy. Check your policy to make sure you are covered and to determine whether there are any limits on what types of reconstruction are covered. Some insurance companies will deny breast reconstruction costs if a claim has been submitted for a form that fits into the bra (an external breast prosthesis); make sure this is not the case with your insurer.

Possible Risks

Any surgery has risks, and reconstruction may pose certain unique problems for some people. These are some of the risks of reconstructive surgery:

- bleeding
- fluid build-up with swelling and pain
- growth of scar tissue
- infection
- tissue death (necrosis) of all or part of the flap, skin, or fat
- problems at the donor site (right away or later on)
- loss of or changes in nipple and breast sensation
- extreme tiredness (fatigue)
- the need for further surgery to fix problems that come up
- changes in the affected arm
- problems with anesthesia

Risks of smoking: Using tobacco causes the blood vessels to constrict (tighten) and reduces the supply of nutrients and oxygen to tissues. Smoking can delay healing, which can cause more noticeable scars and a longer recovery time. Sometimes these problems are bad enough that a second operation is needed to fix them. You may be asked to quit smoking a few weeks or months before surgery to reduce these risks.

Risk of infection: Infection can happen with any surgery, usually in the first 2 weeks after surgery. If an implant has been used, it may have to be removed until the infection clears. A new implant can be put in later. If you have a tissue flap, surgery may be needed to clean the wound.

Risk of capsular contracture: The most common problem with breast implants is **capsular contracture**. This happens when the scar (or capsule) around the implant tightens and starts to squeeze the soft implant. It can make the breast feel very hard. Capsular contracture can be treated. Sometimes surgery can remove the scar tissue, or the implant may be removed or replaced.

Risk of necrosis: Scarring is a natural outcome of any surgery, but cell death (called necrosis) of the breast skin, the flap, or transplanted fat can happen. Immediate reconstruction may be more likely to result in necrosis. If this happens, more surgery is needed to fix the problem and can deform the new breast shape.

After Breast Reconstruction Surgery

What to expect

You are likely to feel tired and sore for a week or two after implants and longer after flap procedures. Your doctor can give you medicines to control pain and other discomfort.

Depending on the type of surgery, you should go home from the hospital in 1 to 6 days. You may be discharged with a drain in place. The drain is an open tube that is left in place to remove extra fluid from the surgery site while it heals. Follow your doctor's instructions on wound and drain care. Also be sure to ask what kind of support garments you should wear. If you have any concerns or questions, call your doctor.

Getting back to normal

You should be up and around in 6 to 8 weeks. If implants are used without flaps, your recovery time may be shorter. Keep these things in mind:

- Reconstruction does not restore normal feeling to your breast, but some feeling may return.
- It may take up to about 8 weeks for bruising and swelling to go away. Try to be patient as you wait to see the final result.
- It may take as long as 1 to 2 years for tissues to heal and scars to fade, but the scars never totally go away.
- Ask when you can go back to wearing regular bras. Underwires and lace may not be comfortable.
- Follow your surgeon's advice on when to begin stretching exercises and normal activities. As a rule, you'll want to avoid any overhead lifting, strenuous sports, and sex for 4 to 6 weeks after reconstruction.
- Women who have reconstruction months or years after a mastectomy may go through a period of emotional readjustment once they have breast reconstruction. Just as it takes time to get used to the loss of a breast, you may feel anxious and confused

as you adjust to the reconstructed breast. Talking with other women who have had breast reconstruction may be helpful. Talking with a mental health professional may also help you sort out these feelings.

- Silicone gel implants may open up or leak inside the body without causing symptoms. Some surgeons will recommend regular MRIs of the implant to make sure it is not leaking. You will likely have your first MRI about a year after your implant surgery and every 2 years from then on. Your insurance may not cover these scans. Talk to your doctor about long-term follow-up.

Studies show that reconstruction does not make breast cancer come back. If the cancer does come back, reconstructed breasts should not cause problems with chemotherapy or radiation treatment. Breast reconstruction rarely, if ever, hides a return of breast cancer. You should not consider recurrence a big risk when deciding whether to have breast reconstruction after mastectomy.

It is important to have regular mammograms on both breasts after reconstruction. If your reconstruction involves an implant, be sure to get your mammograms done at a facility with technologists trained in moving the implant to get the best possible images of the rest of the breast. Pictures can sometimes be impaired by implants, more so by silicone than saline-filled. Reconstructed breasts can look fatty, and surgical clips and scars may show up on the mammogram.

Questions to Ask

What Should You Ask Your Doctor About Breast Cancer?

It is important for you to have open, honest discussions with your doctor about your condition. Do not be afraid to ask questions, no matter how minor they may seem. Here are some questions to consider:

- What type of breast cancer do I have? How does this affect my treatment options and prognosis?
- Has my cancer spread to lymph nodes or internal organs?
- What is the stage of my cancer and how does it affect my treatment options and prognosis?
- Are there other tests that need to be done before we can decide on treatment?
- Should I consider genetic testing?
- Should I think about taking part in a clinical trial?
- What treatments are appropriate for me? What do you recommend? Why?
- What risks and side effects should I expect?
- What do I do if my arm swells?

- How effective will breast reconstruction surgery be if I need or want it?
- What are the advantages and disadvantages of having reconstructive surgery done immediately or waiting until later?
- What will my breasts look and feel like after my treatment? Will I have normal sensation?
- How long will treatment last? What will it involve? Where will it be done?
- What should I do to prepare for treatment?
- Will I need a blood transfusion?
- Should I follow a special diet or make other lifestyle changes?
- What are the chances my cancer will come back after treatment? What would we do if that happens?
- Will I go through menopause as a result of the treatment?
- Will I be able to have children after treatment?
- What type of follow-up care will I need after treatment?

Write down any other questions you have that are not on this list. For instance, you might want specific information about recovery times so that you can plan your work schedule. You might want to ask about second opinions. Taking another person and/or a voice recorder to the appointment is also helpful. Take time to make copies of your medical records, pathology reports, and radiology reports in case you wish to seek a second opinion at a later time.

After Treatment

What Happens After Treatment for Breast Cancer?

Completing treatment can be both stressful and exciting. You will probably be relieved to finish treatment, yet it is hard not to worry about a cancer recurrence (when cancer comes back). The fear of recurrence is very common among people who have had cancer. It may take some time for your fears to lessen and for you to begin to have confidence in your own recovery. Even with no recurrences, people who have had cancer learn to live with uncertainty. For more information on managing these feelings, contact your American Cancer Society at **800-227-2345** and request the document *Living with Uncertainty: The Fear of Cancer Recurrence,* or visit our Web site, **cancer.org**.

Follow-up Care

After treatment is completed, it is very important for you to go to all scheduled follow-up appointments. During these visits, your doctor may ask you questions about any symptoms, perform a physical examination, and order laboratory tests or imaging tests to look for recurrences or side effects. Almost any cancer treatment can have side effects. Some may last for a few weeks to several months, but others can be permanent. Never hesitate to tell your doctor or other members of your cancer care team about any symptoms or side effects that concern you so that they can help you manage them.

At first, your follow-up appointments will probably be scheduled for every 4 to 6 months. The longer you have been free of cancer, the less frequently appointments will be needed. After 5 years, follow-up appointments will typically be done about once a year. If you had breast-conserving surgery, you will need to continue to have mammograms every year.

If you are taking tamoxifen, you should have yearly pelvic exams because this drug can increase your risk of uterine cancer. Contact your doctor right away if you have any abnormal vaginal bleeding. Although vaginal bleeding is usually caused by noncancerous conditions, it could also be the first sign of uterine cancer.

If you are taking an aromatase inhibitor, you may be at increased risk for osteoporosis (thinning of the bones). Your doctor will want to monitor your bone health and may consider testing your bone density.

Other tests such as blood tumor marker studies, blood tests of liver function, bone scans, and chest x-rays are not usually needed unless symptoms or findings from your physical examination suggest the cancer has recurred. However, if you took part in a clinical trial, these and other tests may be done as part of evaluating the new treatments.

If physical examinations and/or tests suggest a recurrence, imaging tests such as an x-ray, CT scan, PET scan, MRI scan, bone scan, or biopsy may be done. Your doctor may also measure the levels of **blood tumor markers** such as CA-15-3, CA 27-29, or CEA (carcinoembryonic antigen) in your blood. If the cancer has spread to bones or other organs such as the liver, the blood levels of these substances will go up in some women. However, blood tumor markers are not elevated in all women with recurrence, so they are not always helpful. If they are elevated, they may help your doctor monitor the results of treatment for the recurrence.

If cancer does recur, the treatment will depend on the location of the cancer and what treatments you have had before. Your treatment may involve surgery, radiation therapy, hormone therapy, chemotherapy, targeted therapy, or some combination of these therapies. For more information on how recurrent cancer is treated, see the section "How Is Breast Cancer Treated?" on pages 185–186. For more general information on dealing with a recurrence, contact your American Cancer Society at **800-227-2345** and request the document *When Your Cancer Comes Back: Cancer Recurrence,* or visit our Web site, **cancer.org**.

Lymphedema

Lymphedema is the swelling of any limb or limb part (such as the hand, wrist, arm, ankle, calf, or leg) due to insufficient drainage of the lymphatic system. It can happen if the person has had lymph nodes removed during surgery or if the person has undergone radiation treatment that has damaged or caused swelling in lymph nodes. Lymphedema can occur at any time after treatment for breast cancer.

One of the first symptoms of lymphedema is a feeling of tightness in the arm or hand on the side of the body that was treated for breast cancer. Any swelling, tightness, or injury to the arm or hand should be reported promptly to your doctor or nurse.

There is no sure way to predict who will get lymphedema. It can develop right after surgery or occur months or even years later. The possibility that lymphedema will develop remains throughout a woman's lifetime. With care, lymphedema can often be avoided or, if it develops, kept under control. Injury or infection involving the affected arm or hand can contribute to the development of lymphedema or worsen existing lymphedema, so preventive measures should focus on protecting the arm and hand. Most doctors recommend that women avoid having their blood pressure taken or having blood drawn from the arm on the side of the body affected by lymph node surgery or radiation. Women should also wear a compression sleeve on the affected arm when traveling by air; a well-fitted compression sleeve may help prevent swelling by helping to squeeze the lymphatic fluid through the remaining vessels before it builds up. To learn more about lymphedema, contact your

American Cancer Society at **800-227-2345** and request the document *Lymphedema: What Every Woman with Breast Cancer Should Know,* or visit our Web site, **cancer.org.**

Quality of Life

Women who have had treatment for breast cancer should be reassured that while they may be left with reminders of their treatment (such as surgical scars), their overall **quality of life** can be normal once treatment is completed. Extensive studies have shown this to be true. Women who have had chemotherapy may notice a slight decrease in certain areas of function.

Some studies suggest that younger women, who represent about 1 of every 4 breast cancer survivors, tend to have more problems adjusting to the stresses of breast cancer and its treatment. They may struggle more with emotional and social functioning. Some can feel isolated. For some younger women, chemotherapy may have caused early menopause, which can be very distressing on its own. There may also be sexual difficulties. These issues may be helped with counseling and support groups for younger breast cancer survivors.

Emotional Aspects of Breast Cancer

Your focus on tests and treatments should not prevent you from considering your emotional, psychological, and spiritual health. Once treatment ends, you may find yourself overwhelmed by emotions. This happens to many people. You may have been going through so much during treatment that you could focus only on getting through your treatment. Now you may find that you think about the potential of your own death or the effect of your cancer on your family, friends, and career. You may also begin to reevaluate your relationship with your spouse or partner. Some unexpected issues can also cause concern—for instance, as you become healthier and have fewer doctor visits, you will see your health care team less often. This change can be a source of anxiety for some people.

This is an ideal time to seek out emotional and social support. You need people you can turn to for strength and comfort. Support can come in many forms: family, friends, cancer support groups, church or spiritual groups, online support communities, or individual counselors. Almost everyone who has been through cancer can benefit from getting some type of support. What is best for you will depend on your situation and your personality. Some people feel safe in peer-support groups or education groups. Others would rather talk in an informal setting, such as at church gatherings. Others may feel more at ease talking one-on-one with a trusted friend or counselor. Whatever your source of strength or comfort, make sure you have a place to go with your concerns.

The cancer journey can feel very lonely. It is not necessary or realistic to go it all by yourself. And your friends and family may feel shut out if you do not include them. Allow them—and anyone else you feel may be able to help—to be there for you. You can also call the American Cancer Society at

800-227-2345 to find out about nearby groups or other resources that can help you as well.

Body Image

Along with having to cope with the emotional stress that cancer and its treatment can cause, many women with breast cancer also find themselves dealing with changes in their appearance as a result of their treatment.

Some changes are short term, such as hair loss. But even short-term changes can have a profound effect on how a woman feels about herself. A number of options are available to help women cope with hair loss, including wigs, hats, scarves, and other accessories. (For a list of companies that sell wigs and other hair accessories, contact your American Cancer Society at **800-227-2345** and request the document *Breast Prostheses and Hair Loss Accessories List,* or visit our Web site, **cancer .org**.) Alternatively, some women may choose to use their baldness as a way to identify themselves as breast cancer survivors.

Other changes that result from breast cancer treatment may be more permanent, such as the loss of part or all of a breast (or breasts) after surgery. Some women may choose reconstructive surgery as a way to deal with this change, others may opt for a breast form, and others may choose to go without any sort of prosthesis.

Regardless of the changes you experience, support is available to help you cope. Speaking with your doctor or other members of your health care team is often a good starting point. There are also many support groups available, such as the American Cancer Society's Reach to Recovery program. Call **800-227-2345** to learn more about programs in your area.

Breast forms and bras vs. breast reconstruction

Following a mastectomy (or, in some cases, breast-conserving surgery), a woman may consider having the breast rebuilt, or reconstructed. Breast reconstruction is usually discussed before surgery to treat the cancer. Decisions about the type of reconstruction and when it will be done depend on each woman's medical situation and personal preferences. Breast reconstruction is discussed in more detail on pages 188–203.

A **breast form** is a prosthesis (artificial body part) worn either inside a bra or attached to the body to simulate the appearance and feel of a natural breast. For women who have had a mastectomy, breast forms can be an important alternative to breast reconstruction. Some women may not want further surgery, knowing that breast reconstruction can sometimes require several procedures to complete.

If you are planning on using a breast form, your doctor will tell you when you have healed enough to be fitted for a permanent breast form or prosthesis. Most of these forms are made from materials that mimic the movement, feel, and weight of natural tissue. A properly weighted breast form provides the balance your body needs for correct posture and anchors your bra, keeping it from riding up.

At first, these forms may feel too heavy, but in time you will adjust to it. Prices vary considerably. A high price does not necessarily mean that the product is the best for you. Take time to shop for a good fit, comfort, and an attractive, natural appearance in the bra and under clothing. Your clothes should fit the way they did before surgery.

The right bra for you may very well be the type you have always worn. It may or may not need adjustments. If there is tenderness while your body is healing, a bra extender can help by increasing the circumference of the bra so that it does not bind the chest too tightly. Large-breasted women can relieve pressure from shoulder straps by slipping a bra shoulder pad under one or both straps.

If you decide to wear the breast form in a pocket in your bra, you can have your regular bra adapted. Special mastectomy bras with pockets already sewn in are also available. If the breast form causes any kind of skin irritation, use a bra with a pocket. If you typically wear an underwire bra, you may be able to continue wearing it, but discuss it with your doctor first.

Some people choose to wear their prosthesis when they sleep and prefer something more comfortable than their regular bra. Most department stores carry a soft bra, sometimes called a leisure bra or night bra.

Insurance coverage of breast prostheses can vary. Be sure to read your insurance policy to determine what is covered and how claims should be submitted. Ask your doctor to write prescriptions for your prosthesis and for any special mastectomy bras. When purchasing bras or breast forms, mark the bills and any checks you write "surgical." Medicare and Medicaid can be used to pay for some of these expenses if you are eligible. The cost of breast forms and bras with pockets may be tax deductible, as may the cost of having a bra altered. Keep careful records of all related expenses.

Some insurance companies will not cover both a breast prosthesis and reconstructive surgery. That can mean that if you submit a claim for a prosthesis or bra to your insurance company, in some cases the company will not cover reconstruction if you choose this procedure in the future. Get all the facts before submitting any insurance claims.

Consider contacting a local American Cancer Society Reach to Recovery volunteer with any questions you have. She will be able to give you suggestions, additional reading material, and advice.

Sexuality

Concerns about sexuality can be very worrisome for a woman with breast cancer. Several factors may place a woman at higher risk for sexual problems after breast cancer. Physical changes (such as those after surgery) may make a woman less comfortable with her body. Some treatments for breast cancer, such as chemotherapy, can change a woman's hormone levels and may negatively affect sexual interest and/or response. A diagnosis of breast cancer when a woman is in her 20s or 30s can be especially difficult because choosing a partner and childbearing are often very important during this period.

Here are some suggestions that can help you adjust to changes in your body:

- Take time to look at and touch your body to become more comfortable.
- Seek the support of others before and after surgery.
- Involve your partner in your recovery as soon as possible.
- Openly communicate the feelings, needs, and wants created by your changed body image.

Sexual impact of surgery and radiation

The most common sexual side effects stem from damage to a woman's feelings of attractiveness. In American culture, we are taught to view breasts as a basic part of beauty and femininity. If her breast has been removed, a woman may be insecure about whether her partner will accept her and find her sexually attractive.

The breasts and nipples are also sources of sexual pleasure for many women. Touching the breasts is a common part of foreplay. For many women, breast stimulation adds to sexual excitement. Treatment for breast cancer can interfere with pleasure from breast caressing. After a mastectomy, the whole breast is gone. Some women still enjoy being stroked around the area of the healed scar. Others dislike being touched there and may no longer even enjoy being touched on the remaining breast and nipple. Some women who have had a mastectomy may feel self-conscious in sexual positions where the area of the missing breast is more visible.

Breast surgery or radiation to the breasts does not physically decrease a woman's sexual desire. Nor does it decrease her ability to have vaginal lubrication or normal genital feelings or to reach orgasm. Recent research indicates that within a year of surgery, most women with early-stage breast cancer have good emotional adjustment and sexual satisfaction. They report a quality of life similar to that of women who never had cancer.

A few women have chronic pain in their chests and shoulders after radical mastectomy. Supporting these areas with pillows during intercourse and avoiding positions where your weight rests on your chest or arms may help.

The breast may be scarred if the woman had breast-conserving therapy. It also may be a different shape or size. During radiation therapy, the skin may become red and swollen. The breast also may be a little tender. These side effects should go away, and feeling in the breast and nipple should return to normal.

Sexual impact of breast reconstruction

Breast reconstruction restores the shape of the breast, but it cannot restore normal breast sensation. The nerve that supplies feeling to the nipple runs through the deep breast tissue, and it is disconnected during mastectomy. In a reconstructed breast, the rebuilt nipple has much less sensation, so the feeling of pleasure from touching the nipple is lost. In time, the skin on the reconstructed breast will regain some sensitivity, though it will probably not give the same kind of pleasure as before a mastectomy. Breast reconstruction often helps women feel more comfortable with their bodies, however, and helps them feel more attractive.

Sexual effects for your partner

Relationship issues are also important because a cancer diagnosis can be very distressing for your partner as well as for you. Your partner may be concerned about how to express his or her love physically and emotionally after treatment, especially after surgery. Breast cancer can be a growth experience for couples under certain circumstances. Your relationship may be enhanced if your partner takes part in decision-making and comes with you to doctor's appointments, surgery, and other treatments.

Pregnancy After Breast Cancer

Because of the well-established link between estrogen levels and growth of breast cancer cells, many doctors advise breast cancer survivors not to become pregnant for at least 2 years after treatment. This delay would allow any early return of the cancer to be diagnosed, which in turn could affect a woman's decision to become pregnant. But this 2-year wait period is not based on strong scientific evidence, and earlier pregnancy may not be harmful. Although few studies have been done, nearly all have found that pregnancy does not increase the risk of recurrence after successful treatment of breast cancer.

Women should discuss their risk of recurrence with their doctors. In some cases, counseling can help women deal with the complex issues and uncertainties of motherhood and breast cancer survivorship.

Postmenopausal Hormone Therapy After Breast Cancer

The known link between estrogen levels and breast cancer growth has discouraged many women and their doctors from choosing or recommending postmenopausal hormone therapy (PHT), also known as hormone replacement therapy (HRT), to help relieve the symptoms of menopause. Unfortunately, many women experience menopausal symptoms after treatment for breast cancer. The onset of symptoms can occur naturally, as a result of postmenopausal women stopping PHT, or in premenopausal women as a result of chemotherapy or ovarian ablation. Tamoxifen can also cause menopausal symptoms such as hot flashes.

In the past, because early studies had shown no harm, doctors often offered PHT after breast cancer treatment to women suffering from severe menopausal symptoms. However, a well-designed clinical trial (the HABITS study) found that breast cancer survivors taking PHT were at much higher risk for a new or recurrent breast cancer than women who were not taking PHT. For this reason, most doctors now feel that PHT is unwise for women who have undergone treatment for breast cancer.

Women should talk with their doctors about alternatives to PHT to help with specific menopausal symptoms. Some doctors have suggested that phytoestrogens (estrogen-like substances from certain plant sources, such as soy products) may be safer than the estrogens used in PHT. However, there is not enough information available on phytoestrogens to fully evaluate their safety for breast cancer survivors.

Drugs without hormonal properties that may be somewhat effective in treating hot flashes include the antidepressant venlafaxine (Effexor), the blood pressure drug clonidine, and the nerve drug gabapentin (Neurontin). Acupuncture also seems to be helpful in treating hot flashes. For women taking tamoxifen (Nolvadex), it is important to note that some antidepressants, known as SSRIs, may interact with tamoxifen and make it less effective. Ask your doctor about possible interactions between tamoxifen and any drugs you may be taking.

Seeing a New Doctor

At some point after your cancer diagnosis and treatment, you may find yourself in the office of a new doctor. Your original doctor may have moved or retired, or you may have moved or changed doctors for some other reason. It is important that you be able to give your new doctor the exact details of your diagnosis and treatment. Make sure you have the following information available:

- a copy of your pathology report(s) from any biopsy or surgery
- a copy of your operative report(s) if you had surgery
- a copy of the discharge summary that doctors must prepare when patients are sent home if you were hospitalized
- a copy of your treatment summary for any radiation therapy you were given
- a list of any other systemic therapies you received (such as hormone therapy, chemotherapy, or targeted therapies), including a list of drugs, drug doses, and when you took them

It is very important that you maintain your medical insurance. Even though no one wants to think that her cancer will come back, it is always a possibility. If you have a recurrence, you will need medical insurance to help you pay for treatment.

Lifestyle Changes to Consider During and After Treatment

You cannot change the fact that you have had cancer. What you can change is how you live the rest of your life—making healthy choices and feeling as well as possible, physically and emotionally. Having cancer and dealing with treatment can be time-consuming and emotionally draining, but it can also be a time to look at your life in new ways.

Make healthier choices

Think about your life before you learned you had cancer. Did you make choices that might have made you less healthy? Maybe you drank too much alcohol, or ate more than you needed, or smoked, or did not exercise very often. Emotionally, maybe you kept your emotions bottled up, or maybe you let stressful situations continue for too long.

Now is not the time to feel guilty or to blame yourself. However, you can start making lifestyle changes today that can help you feel better and improve your health for the long term. What better time than now to take advantage of the motivation you have after going through a life-changing experience like having cancer?

You can start by working to change the habits that concern you the most. Some changes may be difficult, and you should take advantage of any resources available to help you. Get help with those that are harder for you. For instance, if you are thinking about quitting smoking and need help, call the American Cancer Society's Quitline® tobacco cessation program at **800-227-2345**.

Diet and nutrition

Eating right can be a challenge for anyone, but it can become even more difficult during and after cancer treatment. Treatment may change your sense of taste. Nausea can be a problem. You may lose your appetite for a while and lose weight. It is also frustrating for those who instead gain weight, even without eating more.

If you are losing weight or have taste problems during treatment, eat as well as you can and remember that these problems usually improve over time. You may want to ask your doctor for a referral to a registered dietitian, an expert in nutrition who can give you ideas on how to fight some of the side effects of your treatment. You may also find it helps to eat small portions every 2 to 3 hours until you feel better and can return to a more normal eating schedule.

One of the best things you can do after treatment is to establish healthy eating habits. You will be surprised at the long-term benefits of some simple changes, such as increasing the variety of healthy foods you eat. Try to eat 5 or more servings of vegetables and fruits each day. Choose whole grain foods instead of white flour and sugars. Limit or avoid meats that are high in fat and processed meats such as hot dogs, bologna, and bacon. Get rid of them altogether if you can. If you drink alcohol, limit yourself to 1 or 2 drinks a day at the most. Begin exercising regularly. The combination of a good diet and regular exercise will help you maintain a healthy weight and increase your energy level.

Weight

After a breast cancer diagnosis, achieving or maintaining a desirable weight may be one of the most important things you can do. Most studies have found that women who are overweight or obese when their breast cancer is first diagnosed are more likely to have their disease recur and are more likely to die of breast cancer. Overweight women should be encouraged to lose weight after treatment. In some cases, a modest weight loss program can be started during treatment, if the doctor approves.

Study results have been mixed as to how strongly weight gain *after* diagnosis affects breast cancer recurrence or survival. Some studies have found that those who gained significant amounts of weight after diagnosis were more likely to relapse and more likely to die than were women who gained less weight. However, other recent studies have not found that weight gain affected prognosis.

Fatigue, exercise, and rest

Fatigue is a very common side effect of cancer treatment. Cancer-related fatigue is often not an ordinary type of tiredness but a bone-weary exhaustion that does not improve with rest. For some people, this fatigue can last a long time after treatment and can discourage them from physical activity. However, exercise can actually help reduce fatigue. Studies have shown that people who follow an exercise program tailored to their personal needs feel physical and emotional improvement and can cope better.

If you are ill and need to be on bed rest during treatment, it is normal to experience some decline in your fitness, endurance, and muscle strength. Physical therapy can help you maintain your strength and range of motion, which can help fight fatigue and the sense of depression that sometimes comes with fatigue.

Any program of physical activity you undertake should fit your specific situation. An older person who has never exercised will not be able to take on the same amount of exercise as a 20-year-old who is accustomed to playing tennis 3 times a week. If you have not exercised in a few years but are still mobile, you may want to think about taking short walks.

Talk with your health care team and get their opinion before starting an exercise program. Then, recruit a family member or friend to join you. Having an exercise buddy will give you the extra boost of support you need to keep you going when you may not feel as motivated.

If you are very tired, though, you will need to balance activity with rest. It is important that you rest when you need to. It can be hard for people who are used to working all day or taking care of a household to allow themselves to rest, but it is crucial.

Exercise can improve your physical and emotional health in several ways:

- It improves your cardiovascular (heart and circulation) fitness.
- It strengthens your muscles.
- It reduces fatigue.
- It lowers anxiety and depression.
- It makes you feel generally happier.
- It helps you feel better about yourself.

Long term, we know that exercise plays a role in preventing some cancers. The American Cancer Society recommends that to reduce the risk of breast cancer, women should take part in moderate to vigorous physical activity for 45 to 60 minutes on 5 or more days of the week. Moderate physical activities are those that take about as much effort as a brisk walk. Vigorous activities use larger muscle groups, make you sweat, and cause a noticeable increase in heart rate and breathing. The role of physical activity in reducing the risk of breast cancer recurrence is less well defined, although several studies suggest that breast cancer survivors who are physically active may have lower rates of recurrence and death than those who are inactive.

What Happens If Treatment Is No Longer Working?

If cancer continues to grow or return after one kind of treatment, it is often possible to try another treatment plan that might still cure the cancer or shrink the tumors enough to help you live longer and feel better. However, when a person has received several different medical treatments and the cancer has not been cured, over time the cancer tends to become resistant to all treatment. At this time, it is important to weigh the possible limited benefit of a new treatment against the possible disadvantages, including continued doctor visits and treatment side effects.

Each person will have a different way of facing this difficult situation. Some people may want to focus on remaining comfortable during the time they have left. This is likely to be the most difficult time in your battle with cancer—when you have tried every medical treatment within reason and it is just not working anymore. Although your doctor may offer you new treatment, you need to consider that at some point, continuing treatment is not likely to improve your health or change your prognosis for survival.

If you want to continue treatment to fight your cancer for as long as you can, you still need to consider the odds of whether more treatment will have any benefit. In many cases, your doctor can estimate the response rate for the treatment you are considering. Some people are tempted to try more chemotherapy or radiation even if the odds of benefit are less than 1%. In this situation, you need to think about and understand your reasons for choosing this plan.

No matter what you choose, it is important that you be as comfortable as possible. Make sure you are asking for and receiving treatment for any symptoms, such as pain. This type of treatment is called **palliative treatment**. Palliative treatment helps relieve symptoms but is not expected to cure the disease. The main purpose of palliative treatment is to improve your quality of life. Sometimes the treatments used to control your symptoms are similar to the treatments used to treat cancer. For example, radiation therapy might be given to help relieve bone pain from bone metastasis. Chemotherapy could be used to help shrink a tumor and keep it from causing a bowel obstruction. This is not the same as receiving treatment to try to cure the cancer.

At some point, you may benefit from **hospice** care. Most of the time, hospice care is given at home. Your cancer may be causing troublesome symptoms or problems, and hospice focuses on your comfort. Receiving hospice care does not mean you cannot continue treatment for the problems caused by your cancer or other health conditions. The focus of hospice care is to help you live life as fully as possible and feel as well as you can at this difficult stage of your cancer.

Remember also that maintaining hope is important. Your hope for a cure may not be as bright, but there is still hope for good times with family and friends—times that are filled with happiness and meaning. Pausing at this time in your cancer treatment can be an opportunity to refocus on the most important things in your life. This is the time to do some things you have always wanted to do and to stop doing the things you no longer want to do.

Latest Research

What's New in Breast Cancer Research and Treatment?

Research into the causes, prevention, and treatment of breast cancer is now in progress in many medical centers throughout the world.

Causes of Breast Cancer

Studies continue to uncover lifestyle factors and habits that affect breast cancer risk. The effects of exercise, weight gain or loss, and diet on breast cancer risk are all topics of study. Studies on the best use of genetic testing for BRCA1 and BRCA2 mutations continue at a rapid pace. Scientists are also exploring how common gene variations may affect breast cancer risk. Each gene variant has only a modest effect on risk (10% to 20%) but when considered together, they have a potentially large impact.

Potential causes of breast cancer in the environment have also received more attention in recent years. While much of the science on this topic is still in its earliest stages, this is an area of active research.

A large, long-term study funded by the National Institute of Environmental Health Sciences (NIEHS) is now under way to help find the causes of breast cancer. Known as the Sister Study, it has enrolled 50,000 women who have sisters with breast cancer. This study will follow these women for at least 10 years and collect information about genes, lifestyle, and environmental factors that may cause breast cancer. An offshoot of the Sister Study, the Two Sister Study, is designed to look at possible causes of early-onset breast cancer. To find out more about these studies, call 877-4-SISTER (877-474-7837) or visit the Sister Study Web site (www.sisterstudy.org).

Chemoprevention

Results of several studies suggest that selective estrogen-receptor modulators (SERMs), such as tamoxifen and raloxifene, may lower breast cancer risk in women with certain risk factors. However, many women are reluctant to take these medicines because they are concerned about possible side effects.

Newer studies are looking at whether aromatase inhibitors—drugs such as anastrozole, letrozole, and exemestane—can reduce the risk of breast cancer in postmenopausal women. These drugs are already being used as adjuvant hormone therapy to help prevent breast cancer recurrence, but none of them are approved for reducing breast cancer risk at this time.

Fenretinide, a retinoid (a drug related to vitamin A), is also being studied as a way to reduce the risk of breast cancer. In a small study, this drug reduced breast cancer risk as much as tamoxifen. Other drugs are also being studied to reduce the risk of breast cancer. For more information, contact your American Cancer Society at **800-227-2345** and request the document *Medicines to Reduce Breast Cancer Risk,* or visit our Web site, **cancer.org**.

New Laboratory Tests

Gene expression studies

One of the dilemmas with early-stage breast cancer is that doctors cannot always accurately predict which women have a higher risk of recurrence after treatment. That is why most women, except for those with small tumors, usually receive some sort of adjuvant treatment after surgery. Researchers have looked at many aspects of breast cancer to try to better determine who will need adjuvant therapy.

In recent years, scientists have been able to link certain patterns of genes with more aggressive cancers—those that tend to recur and spread to distant sites. Some laboratory tests based on these findings, such as the Oncotype DX and MammaPrint tests, are already available, although doctors are still trying to determine the best way to use them. These tests are explained in the section "How Is Breast Cancer Diagnosed?" on pages 89–90. Other tests are being developed as well.

Classifying breast cancer

Research on patterns of gene expression has also suggested some newer ways of classifying breast cancers. The current types of breast cancer are based largely on how tumors look under a microscope. A newer classification, based on molecular features, may be better able to predict prognosis and response to several types of breast cancer treatment. The new research suggests that there are 4 basic types of breast cancers:

Luminal A and luminal B types: The luminal A and luminal B types are estrogen receptor (ER)–positive, usually have a low grade, and tend to grow fairly slowly. The gene expression patterns of these cancers are similar to those of the normal cells that line the breast ducts and glands (the lining of a duct or gland is called its lumen). Luminal A cancers have the best prognosis. Luminal B cancers usually grow faster than the luminal A cancers, and their prognosis is not quite as favorable.

HER2 type: HER2 type cancers have extra copies of the HER2 gene and several other genes. They usually have a high-grade appearance under the microscope. These cancers tend to grow more quickly and have a worse prognosis, although they often can be treated successfully with targeted therapies such as trastuzumab and lapatinib.

Basal type: Most basal type cancers are of the so-called triple-negative type, meaning they lack estrogen or progesterone receptors and have normal amounts of HER2. The gene expression patterns of these cancers are similar to those of cells in the deeper basal layers of breast ducts and glands. This type is more common among women with BRCA1 gene mutations. For reasons that are not well understood, this type is also more common among younger women and black women.

Basal-type cancers are high-grade cancers that tend to grow quickly and have a poor prognosis. Hormone therapy and anti-HER2 therapies like trastuzumab and lapatinib are not effective against these cancers, although chemotherapy can be helpful. A great deal of research is being done to find better ways to treat these cancers.

It is hoped that these new breast cancer classifications might someday allow doctors to better tailor breast cancer treatments, but more research is needed before this will be possible.

Tests of HER2 status

Determining a breast cancer's HER2 status is important—both to get an idea of how aggressive the cancer is and to find out whether certain drugs that target HER2 can be used to treat the disease. Two types of tests—immunohistochemistry (IHC) and fluorescence in situ hybridization (FISH)—are currently used to determine HER2 status. The FISH test is generally thought to be more accurate, but it also requires special equipment, which can make testing more expensive.

A newer type of test, known as chromogenic in situ hybridization (CISH), works similarly to FISH, by using small DNA probes to count the number of HER2 genes in breast cancer cells. But this test looks for color changes (not fluorescence) and does not require a special microscope, which may make it less expensive. Unlike other tests, CISH can be used on tissue samples that have been stored in the laboratory. Right now, it is not being used as much as IHC or FISH.

Circulating tumor cells

In many women with breast cancer, cancer cells break away from the tumor and enter the blood. These circulating tumor cells can be detected with sensitive laboratory tests. While these tests are not yet available for general use, they may eventually be helpful in determining whether cancer treatment is working or in detecting cancer recurrence after treatment.

Newer Imaging Tests

Several newer imaging methods are now being studied for evaluating abnormalities that may be breast cancers.

Scintimammography

With **scintimammography** (molecular breast imaging), a slightly radioactive substance called technetium sestamibi is injected into a vein. This substance, called a tracer, attaches to breast cancer cells and can be detected by a special camera. Scintimammography is a newer technique that is still being studied to determine whether it is useful in finding breast cancers. Some radiologists believe that it may be helpful in examining suspicious areas found by regular mammograms, but its exact role remains unclear. Current research is aimed at improving the technology and evaluating its use in specific situations, such as in the examination of dense breast tissue in younger women. Some early studies have suggested that it may be almost as accurate as more expensive magnetic resonance imaging (MRI) scans. This test, however, will not replace your usual screening mammogram.

Tomosynthesis

Tomosynthesis (3D mammography) is basically an extension of a digital mammogram. For this test, a woman lies face down on a table with a cut-out hole for the breast, and a machine takes x-rays as it rotates around the breast. Tomosynthesis allows the breast to be viewed as many thin slices, which can be combined into a 3-dimensional picture. It may allow doctors to detect smaller lesions or ones that would otherwise be hidden with standard mammograms. This technology is still considered experimental and is not yet available outside of a clinical trial.

Several other experimental imaging methods, including thermal imaging (thermography), are discussed in the American Cancer Society document *Mammograms and Other Breast Imaging Procedures*. To request a copy of this document, contact your American Cancer Society at **800-227-2345** or visit our Web site, **cancer.org**.

Treatment

Oncoplastic surgery

Breast-conserving surgery (lumpectomy or partial mastectomy) can often be used for early-stage breast cancers. But in some women, these surgeries can result in breasts of different sizes and/or shapes. For larger tumors, breast-conserving surgery might not be possible, and a mastectomy might be needed instead. Some doctors address this problem by combining cancer surgery and plastic surgery, creating a technique known as **oncoplastic surgery**. Oncoplastic surgery typically involves reshaping the breast at the time of the initial breast-conserving surgery and may mean operating on the other breast to make the breasts more symmetrical. This approach is still fairly new, and not all doctors are comfortable with it.

Breast reconstruction surgery

The number of women who are choosing breast-conserving therapy has been steadily increasing. However, there are some women who, for medical or personal reasons, choose to have a mastectomy. Some of them also choose to have reconstructive surgery to restore the breast's appearance.

Technical advances in microvascular surgery (reattaching blood vessels) have made free-flap procedures an option for breast reconstruction. For more information on the types of reconstructive surgery now available, contact your American

Cancer Society at **800-227-2345** and request the document *Breast Reconstruction After Mastectomy,* or visit our Web site, **cancer.org**.

For several years, concern over a possible link between breast implants and immune system diseases has discouraged some women from choosing implants as a method of breast reconstruction. Recent studies have found that although implants can cause some side effects (such as firm or hard scar tissue formation), women with implants are not at greater risk for immune system diseases compared with women who have not had this surgery. Similarly, the concern that breast implants increase the risk of breast cancer recurrence or the formation of new cancers is not supported by current evidence.

Radiation therapy

For women who need radiation therapy after breast-conserving surgery, newer techniques such as hypofractionated radiation or accelerated partial breast irradiation may be as effective as standard radiation therapy, while also offering a more convenient way to receive it (as opposed to the standard weeks-long, daily radiation regimen). These techniques are described in more detail in the section "How Is Breast Cancer Treated?" on pages 138–142. Large studies are being done to determine whether these techniques are as effective as standard radiation in helping prevent cancer recurrences.

New chemotherapy drugs

Because advanced breast cancers are often difficult to treat, researchers are always looking for newer and more effective drugs. One new drug, olaparib, targets cancers caused by BRCA mutations. Olaparib was shown to be successful in treating breast, ovarian, and prostate cancers that had spread and were resistant to other treatments. Further studies are under way to determine whether this drug can help patients without BRCA mutations.

Targeted therapies

Targeted therapies are a group of newer drugs that specifically target gene changes in cells that cause cancer.

Drugs that target HER2: Two drugs have been approved to target excess HER2 protein: trastuzumab (Herceptin) and lapatinib (Tykerb). Studies are continuing to determine which of these drugs is best for early treatment of breast cancer. Other drugs that target the HER2 protein, including pertuzumab and neratinib, are being tested in clinical trials. Researchers are also considering a vaccine to target the HER2 protein.

Antiangiogenesis drugs: In order for cancers to grow, blood vessels must develop to nourish the cancer cells. This process is called angiogenesis. Looking at angiogenesis in breast cancer specimens can help predict prognosis. Some studies have found that breast cancers surrounded by many new, small blood vessels are likely to be more aggressive. More research is needed to confirm this finding.

Bevacizumab is an example of an antiangiogenesis drug. Although the value of this drug for breast cancer is currently uncertain, clinical trials are being done to test several other antiangiogenesis drugs.

Drugs that target the epidermal growth factor receptor: The epidermal growth factor receptor (EGFR) is another protein found in high amounts on the surface of some cancer cells. Some drugs that target EGFR, such as cetuximab and erlotinib, are already used to treat other types of cancers, whereas other anti-EGFR drugs are still considered experimental. Studies are under way to determine whether these drugs might be effective against breast cancer.

Other targeted drugs: Everolimus (Afinitor) is a new type of targeted therapy that was recently approved to treat kidney cancer. In one study, letrozole plus everolimus worked better than letrozole alone in shrinking breast tumors before surgery. More studies using this drug are planned.

Many other potential targets for new breast cancer drugs have been identified in recent years. Drugs based on these targets are now being studied, although most are still in the early stages of clinical trials.

Bisphosphonates

Bisphosphonates are drugs that help strengthen and reduce the risk of fractures in bones that have been weakened by metastatic breast cancer. Examples include pamidronate (Aredia) and zoledronic acid (Zometa).

Some studies have suggested that zoledronic acid may help other systemic therapies, such as hormone treatment and chemotherapy, work better. In one study, more of the women who received zoledronic acid along with chemotherapy had their tumors shrink, as compared with the women who received chemotherapy alone. In other studies, zoledronic acid reduced the risk of cancer recurrence. More studies are needed to determine whether bisphosphonates should become part of standard therapy for early-stage breast cancer.

Vitamin D

A recent study found that women with early-stage breast cancer who were deficient in vitamin D were more likely to have their cancer recur in a distant part of the body and had a less favorable prognosis. More research is needed to confirm this finding, and it is not yet clear whether taking vitamin D supplements would be helpful for women with early-stage breast cancer. You may want to talk to your doctor about testing your vitamin D level to see whether it is in the healthy range.

Denosumab

When cancer spreads to the bone, it causes an increase in the levels of a substance called RANKL, which is important in bone metabolism. Higher levels of RANKL stimulate cells called **osteoclasts** to destroy bone. A newer drug called denosumab acts against RANKL and can help protect bones. In early studies, it seems to have a benefit even when bisphosphanates have stopped working. More studies are ongoing.

Resources

More Information from Your American Cancer Society

No matter who you are, we can help. Contact us anytime, day or night, for information and support. Call us at **800-227-2345** or visit **cancer.org**.

These related documents may also be helpful to you. These materials may be ordered, free of charge, by calling our toll-free number, **800-227-2345**.

After Diagnosis: A Guide for Patients and Families (also available in Spanish)

Bone Metastasis

Breast Cancer Dictionary (also available in Spanish)

Breast Cancer Early Detection (also available in Spanish)

Breast Cancer in Men

Breast Prostheses and Hair Loss Accessories List

Breast Reconstruction After Mastectomy (also available in Spanish)

Chemo Brain

Clinical Trials: What You Need to Know

DES Exposure: Questions and Answers

Exercises After Breast Surgery (also available in Spanish)

Fatigue in People with Cancer

Genetic Testing: What You Need to Know

Inflammatory Breast Cancer

Is Having an Abortion Linked to Breast Cancer?

Living With Uncertainty: The Fear of Cancer Recurrence

Lymphedema: What Every Woman with Breast Cancer Should Know

Mammograms and Other Breast Imaging Procedures

Medicines to Reduce Breast Cancer Risk

Non-cancerous Breast Conditions (also available in Spanish)

Pregnancy and Breast Cancer

Reach to Recovery (also available in Spanish)

Sarcoma—Adult Soft Tissue Cancer

Sexuality for the Woman with Cancer (also available in Spanish)

Talking with Your Doctor (also available in Spanish)

Understanding Chemotherapy (also available in Spanish)

Understanding Radiation Therapy (also available in Spanish)

When Your Cancer Comes Back: Cancer Recurrence

The following books are available from the American Cancer Society. Call us at **800-227-2345** to ask about costs or to place your order. For a full listing of books published by the American Cancer Society, see the list at the end of the book.

American Cancer Society Complete Guide to Nutrition for Cancer Survivors: Eating Well, Staying Well During and After Cancer

Breast Cancer Clear and Simple: All Your Questions Answered

Cancer Caregiving A to Z: An At-Home Guide for Patients and Families

Caregiving: A Step-By-Step Resource for Caring for the Person with Cancer at Home

Couples Confronting Cancer

Lymphedema: Understanding and Managing Lymphedema After Cancer Treatment

Quick Facts: Advanced Cancer

Quick Facts: Bone Metastasis

What to Eat During Cancer Treatment: 100 Great-Tasting, Family-Friendly Recipes to Help You Cope

What Helped Get Me Through: Cancer Survivors Share Wisdom and Hope

National Organizations and Web Sites*

The following organizations can provide additional information and resources:

American Society of Plastic Surgeons (ASPS)
Web site: www.plasticsurgery.org

Breast Cancer Network of Strength (formerly Y-Me National Breast Cancer Organization)
Toll-free number: 800-221-2141, 1-800-986-9505 (Spanish)
Web site: www.networkofstrength.org

Centers for Disease Control and Prevention (CDC)
Toll-free number: 800-232-4636
Web site: www.cdc.gov

Food and Drug Administration Consumer Information Line
Toll-free number: 888-463-6332

---

*Inclusion on this list does not imply endorsement by the American Cancer Society.

Web site: www.fda.gov or www.fda.gov/cdrh/breastimplants

National Breast Cancer Coalition
Toll-free number: 800-622-2838
Web site: www.stopbreastcancer.org

National Cancer Institute
Toll-free number: 800-4-CANCER (1-800-422-6237)
Web site: www.cancer.gov

SHARE: Self-Help for Women with Breast or Ovarian Cancer
Toll-free number: 866-891-2392
Web site: www.sharecancersupport.org

Susan G. Komen for the Cure
Toll-free number: 877-465-6636
Web site: www.komen.org

References

Abeloff MD, Wolff AC, Weber BL, et al. Cancer of the breast. In: Abeloff MD, Armitage JO, Neiderhuber JE, Kastan MB, McKenna WG, eds. *Clinical Oncology*. 4th ed. Philadelphia: Churchill Livingstone/Elsevier; 2008:1875–1943.

Altekruse SF, Kosary CL, Krapcho M, Neyman N, Aminou R, Waldron W, Ruhl J, Howlader N, Tatalovich Z, Cho H, Mariotto A, Eisner MP, Lewis DR, Cronin K, Chen HS, Feuer EJ, Stinchcomb DG, Edwards BK (eds). SEER Cancer Statistics Review, 1975-2007, National Cancer Institute. Bethesda, MD, http://seer.cancer.gov/csr/1975_2007/, based on November 2009 SEER data submission, posted to the SEER web site, 2010.

American Cancer Society. *Cancer Facts and Figures 2010*. Atlanta: American Cancer Society; 2010.

American Joint Committee on Cancer. Breast. In: *AJCC Cancer Staging Manual*. 7th ed. New York: Springer; 2010:347–369.

Avis NE, Crawford S, Manuel J. Quality of life among younger women with breast cancer. *J Clin Oncol*. 2005;23(15):3322–3330.

Barthelmes L, Davidson LA, Gaffney C, Gateley CA. Pregnancy and breast cancer. *BMJ*. 2005;330(7504):1375–1378.

Baselga J, Gelmon KA, Verma S, Wardley A, Conte P, Miles D, Bianchi G, Cortes J, McNally VA, Ross GA, Fumoleau P, Gianni L. Phase II trial of pertuzumab and trastuzumab in patients with human epidermal growth factor receptor 2-positive metastatic breast cancer that progressed during prior trastuzumab therapy. *J Clin Oncol*. 2010;28(7):1138–1144. Epub 2010 Feb 1.

Beral V, Million Women Study Collaborators. Breast cancer and hormone-replacement therapy in the Million Women Study. *Lancet.* 2003;362(9382):419–427.

Erratum in: *Lancet.* 2003;362(9390):1160.

Bohlius J, Wilson J, Seidenfeld J, Piper M, Schwarzer G, Sandercock J, Trelle S, Weingart O, Bayliss S, Djulbegovic B, Bennett CL, Langensiepen S, Hyde C, Engert A. Recombinant human erythropoietins and cancer patients: updated meta-analysis of 57 studies including 9353 patients. *J Natl Cancer Inst.* 2006;98(10):708–714.

Blackwell KL, Burstein HJ, Storniolo AM, Rugo H, Sledge G, Koehler M, Ellis C, Casey M, Vukelja S, Bischoff J, Baselga J, O'Shaughnessy J. Randomized study of lapatinib alone or in combination with trastuzumab in women with ErbB2-positive, trastuzumab-refractory metastatic breast cancer. *J Clin Oncol.* 2010;28(7):1124–1130. Epub 2010 Feb 1.

Brenton JD, Carey LA, Ahmed AA, Caldas C. Molecular classification and molecular forecasting of breast cancer: ready for clinical application? *J Clin Oncol.* 2005;23(29):7350–7360. Epub 2005 Sep 6.

Briot K, Tubiana-Hulin M, Bastit L, Kloos I, Roux C. Effect of a switch of aromatase inhibitors on musculoskeletal symptoms in postmenopausal women with hormone-receptor-positive breast cancer: the ATOLL (articular tolerance of letrozole) study. *Breast Cancer Res Treat.* 2010;120(1):127–134. Epub 2009 Dec 25.

Burstein HJ, Harris JR, Morrow M. Malignant tumors of the breast. In: DeVita VT, Lawrence TS, Rosenberg SA, eds. *DeVita, Hellman, and Rosenberg's Cancer: Principles and Practice of Oncology.* 8th ed. Philadelphia: Lippincott Williams & Wilkins; 2008:1606–1654.

Burstein HJ, Sun Y, Dirix LY, Jiang Z, Paridaens R, Tan AR, Awada A, Ranade A, Jiao S, Schwartz G, Abbas

R, Powell C, Turnbull K, Vermette J, Zacharchuk C, Badwe R. Neratinib, an irreversible ErbB receptor tyrosine kinase inhibitor, in patients with advanced ErbB2-positive breast cancer. *J Clin Oncol.* 2010;28(8):1301–1307. Epub 2010 Feb 8.

Chen CL, Weiss NS, Newcomb P, Barlow W, White E. Hormone replacement therapy in relation to breast cancer. *JAMA.*2002;287(6):734–741.

Chung AP, Sacchini V. Nipple-sparing mastectomy: where are we now? *Surg Oncol.* 2008;17(4):261–266. Erratum in: *Surg Oncol.*2010;19(2):114.

Citron ML, Berry DA, Cirrincione C, Hudis C, Winer EP, Gradishar WJ, Davidson NE, Martino S, Livingston R, Ingle JN, Perez EA, Carpenter J, Hurd D, Hollad JF, Smith BL, Sartor CI, Leung EH, Abrams J, Schilsky RL, Muss HB, Norton L. Randomized trial of dose-dense versus conventionally scheduled and sequential versus concurrent combination chemotherapy as postoperative adjuvant treatment of node-positive primary breast cancer: first report of Intergroup Trial C9741/Cancer and Leukemia Group B Trial 9741. *J Clin Oncol.* 2003;21(8):1431–1439. Epub 2003 Feb 13.
Erratum in: *J Clin Oncol.* 2003;21(8):1425–1428.

Clarke M, Collins R, Darby S, Davies C, Elphinstone P, Evans E, Godwin J, Gray R, Hicks C, James S, MacKinnon E, McGale P, McHugh T, Peto R, Taylor C, Wang Y; Early Breast Cancer Trialists' Collaborative Group (EBCTCG). Effects of radiotherapy and of differences in the extent of surgery for early breast cancer on local recurrence and 15-year survival: an overview of the randomised trials. *Lancet.* 2005;366(9503):2087–2106.

Coleman RE, Winter MC, Cameron D, Bell R, Dodwell D, Keane MM, Gil M, Ritchie D, Passos-Coelho JL, Wheatley D, Burkinshaw R, Marshall SJ,

Thorpe H; AZURE (BIG01/04) Investigators. The effects of adding zoledronic acid to neoadjuvant chemotherapy on tumour response: exploratory evidence for direct anti-tumour activity in breast cancer. *Br J Cancer*. 2010;102(7):1099–1105. Epub 2010 Mar 16.

Collaborative Group on Hormonal Factors in Breast Cancer. Familial breast cancer: collaborative reanalysis of individual data from 52 epidemiological studies including 58,209 women with breast cancer and 101,986 women without the disease. *Lancet*. 2001;358:1389–1399.

Darbre PD, Aljarrah A, Miller WR, Coldham NG, Sauer MJ, Pope GS. Concentrations of parabens in human breast tumours. *J Appl Toxicol*. 2004;24(1):5–13.

Dorval M, Guay S, Mondor M, Mâsse B, Falardeau M, Robidoux A, Deschênes L, Maunsell E. Couples who get closer after breast cancer: frequency and predictors in a prospective investigation. *J Clin Oncol*. 2005;23(15):3588–3596.

Early Breast Cancer Trialists' Collaborative Group (EBCTCG). Effects of chemotherapy and hormonal therapy for early breast cancer on recurrence and 15-year survival: an overview of the randomised trials. *Lancet*. 2005;365(9472):1687–1717.

Fenton JJ, Taplin SH, Carney PA, Abraham L, Sickles EA, D'Orsi C, Berns EA, Cutter G, Hendrick RE, Barlow WE, Elmore JG. Influence of computer-aided detection on performance of screening mammography. *N Engl J Med*. 2007;356(14):1399–1409.

Fisher B, Costantino JP, Wickerham DL, Cecchini RS, Cronin WM, Robidoux A, Bevers TB, Kavanah MT, Atkins JN, Margolese RG, Runowicz CD, James JM, Ford LG, Wolmark N. Tamoxifen for the prevention of breast cancer: current status of the National Surgical Adjuvant Breast and Bowel Project P-1 study. *J Natl Cancer Inst*. 2005;97(22):1652–1662.

Fizazi K, Lipton A, Mariette X, Body JJ, Rahim Y, Gralow JR, Gao G, Wu L, Sohn W, Jun S. Randomized phase II trial of denosumab in patients with bone metastases from prostate cancer, breast cancer, or other neoplasms after intravenous bisphosphonates. *J Clin Oncol*. 2009;27(10):1564–1571. Epub 2009 Feb 23.

Fong PC, Boss DS, Yap TA, Tutt A, Wu P, Mergui-Roelvink M, Mortimer P, Swaisland H, Lau A, O'Connor MJ, Ashworth A, Carmichael J, Kaye SB, Schellens JH, de Bono JS. Inhibition of poly(ADP-ribose) polymerase in tumors from BRCA mutation carriers. *N Engl J Med*. 2009;361(2):123–134. Epub 2009 Jun 24.

Gnant M, Mlineritsch B, Luschin-Ebengreuth G, Kainberger F, Kässmann H, Piswanger-Sölkner JC, Seifert M, Ploner F, Menzel C, Dubsky P, Fitzal F, Bjelic-Radisic V, Steger G, Greil R, Marth C, Kubista E, Samonigg H, Wohlmuth P, Mittlböck M, Jakesz R; Austrian Breast and Colorectal Cancer Study Group (ABCSG). Adjuvant endocrine therapy plus zoledronic acid in premenopausal women with early-stage breast cancer: 5-year follow-up of the ABCSG-12 bone-mineral density substudy. *Lancet Oncol*. 2008;9(9):840–849. Epub 2008 Aug 19.

Goodwin PJ, Ennis M, Pritchard KI, Koo J, Hood N. Prognostic effects of 25-hydroxyvitamin D levels in early breast cancer. *J Clin Oncol*. 2009;27(23)3757–3763. Epub 2009 May 18.

Graeser MK, Engel C, Rhiem K, Gadzicki D, Bick U, Kast K, Froster UG, Schlehe B, Bechtold A, Arnold N, Preisler-Adams S, Nestle-Kraemling C, Zaino M, Loeffler M, Kiechle M, Meindl A, Varga D, Schmutzler RK. Contralateral breast cancer risk in BRCA1 and BRCA2 mutation carriers. *J Clin Oncol*. 2009;27(35):5862–5864.

Holmberg L, Anderson H; HABITS steering and data monitoring committees. HABITS (hormonal replacement therapy after breast cancer—is it safe?), a randomised comparison: trial stopped. *Lancet.* 2004;363(9407):453–455.

Holmes MD, Chen WY, Feskanich D, Kroenke CH, Colditz GA. Physical activity and survival after breast cancer diagnosis. *JAMA.* 2005;293(20):2479–2486.

Horner MJ, Ries LAG, Krapcho M, Neyman N, Aminou R, Howlader N, Altekruse SF, Feuer EJ, Huang L, Mariotto A, Miller BA, Lewis DR, Eisner MP, Stinchcomb DG, Edwards BK, eds. *SEER Cancer Statistics Review, 1975-2006*, National Cancer Institute. Bethesda, MD, http://seer.cancer .gov/csr/1975_2006/, based on November 2008 SEER data submission, posted to the SEER web site, 2009.

Houssami N, Hayes DF. Review of preoperative magnetic resonance imaging (MRI) in breast cancer: should MRI be performed on all women with newly diagnosed, early stage breast cancer? *CA Cancer J Clin.* 2009;59(5):290-302. Epub 2009 Aug 13.

Hudis C, Tan LK. Rare cancers in the breast. In: Harris JR, Lippman ME, Morrow M, Osborne CK, eds. *Diseases of the Breast.* 3rd ed. Philadelphia: Lippincott Williams & Wilkins; 2005:1015–1033.

Joensuu H, Kellokumpu-Lehtinen PL, Bono P, Alanko T, Kataja V, Asola R, Utriainen T, Kokko R, Hemminki A, Tarkkanen M, Turpeenniemi-Hujanen T, Jyrkkiö S, Flander M, Helle L, Ingalsuo S, Johansson K, Jääskeläinen AS, Pajunen M, Rauhala M, Kaleva-Kerola J, Salminen T, Leinonen M, Elomaa I, Isola J; FinHer Study Investigators. Adjuvant docetaxel or vinorelbine with or without trastuzumab for breast cancer. *N Engl J Med.* 2006;354(8):809–820.

Kabat GC, Cross AJ, Park Y, Schatzkin A, Hollenbeck AR, Rohan TE, Sinha R. Meat intake and meat preparation in relation to risk of postmenopausal breast cancer in the NIH-AARP diet and health study. *Int J Cancer*. 2009;124(10):2430–2435.

Kabat GC, Kim M, Adams-Campbell LL, Caan BJ, Chlebowski RT, Neuhouser ML, Shikany JM, Rohan TE; WHI Investigators. Longitudinal study of serum carotenoid, retinol, and tocopherol concentrations in relation to breast cancer risk among postmenopausal women. *Am J Clin Nutr*. 2009;90(1):162–169.

Kushi LH, Byers T, Doyle C, Bandera EV, McCullough M, McTiernan A, Gansler T, Andrews KS, Thun MJ; American Cancer Society 2006 Nutrition and Physical Activity Guidelines Advisory Committee. American Cancer Society guidelines on nutrition and physical activity for cancer prevention: reducing the risk of cancer with healthy food choices and physical activity. *CA Cancer J Clin*. 2006;56(5):254–281; quiz 313–314.

Lawenda BD, Mondry TE, Johnstone PA. Lymphedema: a primer on the identification and management of a chronic condition in oncologic treatment. *CA Cancer J Clin*. 2009;59(1):8–24.

McCloskey E, Paterson A, Kanis J, Tähtelä R, Powles T. Effect of oral clodronate on bone mass, bone turnover and subsequent metastases in women with primary breast cancer. *Eur J Cancer*. 2010;46(3):558–565. Epub 2009 Dec 22.

McTiernan A, Kooperberg C, White E, Wilcox S, Coates R, Adams-Campbell LL, Woods N, Ockene J; Women's Health Initiative Cohort Study. Recreational physical activity and the risk of breast cancer in postmenopausal women: the Women's Health Initiative Cohort Study. *JAMA*. 2003;290(10):1331–1336.

Miles DW, Chan A, Dirix LY, Cortés J, Pivot X, Tomczak P, Delozier T, Sohn JH, Provencher L, Puglisi F, Harbeck N, Steger GG, Schneeweiss A, Wardley AM,

Chlistalla A, Romieu G. Phase III study of bevacizumab plus docetaxel compared with placebo plus docetaxel for the first-line treatment of human epidermal growth factor receptor 2-negative metastatic breast cancer. *J Clin Oncol.* 2010;28(20):3239–3247.

Mirick DK, Davis S, Thomas DB. Antiperspirant use and the risk of breast cancer. *J Natl Cancer Inst.* 2002;94(20):1578–1580.

Morrow M, Strom EA, Bassett LW, Dershaw DD, Fowble B, Harris JR, O'Malley F, Schnitt SJ, Singletary SE, Winchester DP; American College of Surgeons; College of American Pathology; Society of Surgical Oncology; American College of Radiology. Standard for the management of ductal carcinoma in situ of the breast (DCIS). *CA Cancer J Clin.* 2002;52(5):256–276.

National Comprehensive Cancer Network (NCCN). *Practice Guidelines in Oncology: Breast Cancer.* Version 2.2010. Accessed at www.nccn.org on May 20, 2010.

Nattinger AB. Variation in the choice of breast-conserving surgery or mastectomy: patient or physician decision making? *J Clin Oncol.* 2005;23(24):5429–5431.

Nitz UA, Mohrmann S, Fischer J, Lindemann W, Berdel WE, Jackisch C, Werner C, Ziske C, Kirchner H, Metzner B, Souchon R, Ruffert U, Schütt G, Pollmanns A, Schmoll HJ, Middecke C, Baltzer J, Schrader I, Wiebringhaus H, Ko Y, Rösel S, Schwenzer T, Wernet P, Hinke A, Bender HG, Frick M; West German Study Group. Comparison of rapidly cycled tandem high-dose chemotherapy plus peripheral-blood stem-cell support versus dose-dense conventional chemotherapy for adjuvant treatment of high-risk breast cancer: results of a multicentre phase III trial. *Lancet.*

2005;366(9501):1935–1944.
Erratum in: *Lancet.* 2006;367(9512):730.

Olsson HL, Ingvar C, Bladström A. Hormone replacement therapy containing progestins and given continuously increases breast carcinoma risk in Sweden. *Cancer.* 2003;97(6):1387–1392.

Patil R, Clifton GT, Holmes JP, Amin A, Carmichael MG, Gates JD, Benavides LH, Hueman MT, Ponniah S, Peoples GE. Clinical and immunologic responses of HLA-A3+ breast cancer patients vaccinated with the HER2/neu-derived peptide vaccine, E75, in a phase I/II clinical trial. *J Am Coll Surg.* 2010;210(2):140–147. Epub 2009 Dec 22.

Pisano ED, Gatsonis C, Hendrick E, Yaffe M, Baum JK, Acharyya S, Conant EF, Fajardo LL, Bassett L, D'Orsi C, Jong R, Rebner M; Digital Mammographic Imaging Screening Trial (DMIST) Investigators Group. Diagnostic performance of digital versus film mammography for breast-cancer screening. *N Engl J Med.* 2005;353(17):1773–1783.

Rakha EA, Reis-Filho JS, Ellis IO. Basal-like breast cancer: a critical review. *J Clin Oncol.* 2008;26(15):2568–2581.

Rebbeck TR, Lynch HT, Neuhausen SL, Narod SA, Van't Veer L, Garber JE, Evans G, Isaacs C, Daly MB, Matloff E, Olopade OI, Weber BL; Prevention and Observation of Surgical End Points Study Group. Prophylactic oophorectomy in carriers of BRCA1 or BRCA2 mutations. *N Engl J Med.* 2002;346(21):1616–1622.

Ries LAG, Eisner MP. Cancer of the female breast. In: Ries LAG, Young JL, Keel GE, Eisner MP, Lin YD, Horner M-J, eds. *SEER Survival Monograph: Cancer Survival Among Adults: U.S. SEER Program, 1988-2001, Patient and Tumor Characteristics.* Bethesda, MD: National Cancer Institute, SEER Program;

2007:NIH Pub. No. 07-6215. http://seer.cancer.gov/publications/survival. Accessed July 9, 2008.

Robert NJ, Dieras V, Glaspy J, Brufsky A, Bondarenko I, Lipatov O, Perez E, Yardley D, Zhou X, Phan S. RIBBON-1: randomized, double-blind, placebo-controlled, phase III trial of chemotherapy with or without bevacizumab (B) for first-line treatment of HER2-negative locally recurrent or metastatic breast cancer (MBC). *J Clin Oncol*. 2009;27(Suppl):15s. (Abstr 1005).

Ross JS, Hatzis C, Symmans WF, Pusztai L, Hortobágyi GN. Commercialized multigene predictors of clinical outcome for breast cancer. *Oncologist*. 2008;13(5):477–493.
    Erratum in: *Oncologist*. 2008;13(8). doi:10.1634/theoncologist. 2007-0248.

Saslow D, Boetes C, Burke W, Harms S, Leach MO, Lehman CD, Morris E, Pisano E, Schnall M, Sener S, Smith RA, Warner E, Yaffe M, Andrews KS, Russell CA for the American Cancer Society Breast Cancer Advisory Group. American Cancer Society guidelines for breast screening with MRI as an adjunct to mammography. *CA Cancer J Clin*. 2007;57(2):75-89. http://caonline.amcancersoc.org/cgi/content/full/57/2/75. Accessed May 25, 2010.

Thompson D, Easton DF; Breast Cancer Linkage Consortium. Cancer incidence in BRCA1 mutation carriers. *J Natl Cancer Inst*. 2002;94(18):1358–1365.

U.S. Preventive Services Task Force. Genetic risk assessment and BRCA mutation testing for breast and ovarian cancer susceptibility: recommendation statement. *Ann Intern Med*. 2005;143(5):355–361.
    Erratum in: *Ann Intern Med*. 2005;143(7):547.

Untch M, Möbus V, Kuhn W, Muck BR, Thomssen C, Bauerfeind I, Harbeck N, Werner C, Lebeau A, Schneeweiss A, Kahlert S, von Koch F, Petry KU,

Wallwiener D, Kreienberg R, Albert US, Lück HJ, Hinke A, Jänicke F, Konecny GE. Intensive dose-dense compared with conventionally scheduled preoperative chemotherapy for high-risk primary breast cancer. *J Clin Oncol.* 2009;27(18):2938-2945. Epub 2009 Apr 13.

Vadivelu N, Schreck M, Lopez J, Kodumudi G, Narayan D. Pain after mastectomy and breast reconstruction. *Am Surg.* 2008;74(4)285–296.

Vilholm OJ, Cold S, Rasmussen L, Sindrup SH. The postmastectomy pain syndrome: An epidemiological study on the prevalence of chronic pain after surgery for breast cancer. *Br J Cancer.* 2008;99(4):604–610.

Vogel VG, Costantino JP, Wickerham DL, Cronin WM, Cecchini RS, Atkins JN, Bevers TB, Fehrenbacher L, Pajon ER, Wade JL 3rd, Robidoux A, Margolese RG, James J, Runowicz CD, Ganz PA, Reis SE, McCaskill-Stevens W, Ford LG, Jordan VC, Wolmark N; National Surgical Adjuvant Breast and Bowel Project. Update of the National Surgical Adjuvant Breast and Bowel Project Study of Tamoxifen and Raloxifene (STAR) P-2 Trial. Preventing breast cancer. *Cancer Prev Res.* 2010;3(6):696–706. Epub 2010 Apr 19.

Walker EM, Rodriguez AI, Kohn B, Ball RM, Pegg J, Pocock JR, Nunez R, Peterson E, Jakary S, Levine RA. Acupuncture versus venlafaxine for the management of vasomotor symptoms in patients with hormone receptor-positive breast cancer: a randomized controlled trial. *J Clin Oncol.* 2010;28(4):634–640.

Whelan T, MacKenzie R, Julian J, Levine M, Shelley W, Grimard L, Lada B, Lukka H, Perera F, Fyles A, Laukkanen E, Gulavita S, Benk V, Szechtman B. Randomized trial of breast irradiation schedules after lumpectomy for women with lymph node-negative breast cancer. *J Natl Cancer Inst.* 2002;94(15):1143–1150.

Winer EP, Carey LA, Dowsett M, Tripathy D. Beyond anatomic staging: Are we ready to take the leap to molecular classification? In: Perry MC, Whippen D; American Society of Clinical Oncology. *American Society of Clinical Oncology Educational Book.* Alexandria, VA: American Society of Clinical Oncology; 2005.

Glossary

accelerated breast irradiation: *see* external beam radiation therapy (EBRT).

adenocarcinoma (add-uh-no-kahr-si-NO-muh): cancer of the glandular tissue, such as in the ducts or lobules of the breast. *See* duct, lobules.

adjuvant (AJ-uh-vunt) therapy: treatment used in addition to the main treatment. It usually refers to hormone therapy, chemotherapy, radiation therapy, or immunotherapy added after surgery to increase the chances of curing the disease or prevent it from recurring.

alternative therapy (alternative medicine): an unproven medication or therapy that is recommended instead of standard (proven) therapy. Some alternative therapies have dangerous or even life-threatening side effects. With others, the main danger is that the patient may lose the opportunity to benefit from standard therapy. The American Cancer Society recommends that patients considering the use of any alternative or complementary therapies discuss them with their cancer care team. *Compare with* complementary therapy.

American Joint Committee on Cancer (AJCC) staging system: a system for describing the extent of a cancer's spread by using Roman numerals from 0 through IV. Also called the TNM system. *See also* staging.

anesthesia (an-es-THEE-zhuh): the loss of feeling or sensation as a result of drugs or gases. General anesthesia causes loss of consciousness (puts you to sleep). Local or regional anesthesia numbs only a certain area of the body.

anesthetic (an-es-THEH-tik): a topical or intravenous substance that causes loss of feeling or awareness in a part of the body. General anesthetics are used to put patients to sleep for procedures. *See also* anesthesia.

aneuploid (AN-you-ploid): *see* ploidy.

angiogenesis (an-jee-o-JEN-uh-sis): the formation of new blood vessels. Some cancer treatments work by blocking angiogenesis, thus preventing blood from reaching the tumor.

angiosarcoma (AN-jee-o-sar-KO-ma): a type of cancer that begins in the cells that line blood vessels or lymph vessels. Cancer that begins in blood vessels is called hemangiosarcoma. Cancer that begins in lymph vessels is called lymphangiosarcoma.

antibody: a protein produced by the immune system cells and released into the blood. Antibodies defend the body against foreign agents, such as bacteria. These agents contain antigens. Each antibody works against a specific antigen. *See* antigen.

antigen (an-tuh-jin): a substance that causes the body's immune system to respond. This response often involves making antibodies. For example, the immune system's response to antigens that are part of bacteria and viruses helps people resist infections. Cancer cells have certain antigens that can be found in lab tests. These antigens are important in cancer diagnosis and in watching response to treatment. Other antigens play a role in the body's resistance to cancer.

areola (a-REE-o-la): the area of dark-colored skin on the breast that surrounds the nipple.

aromatase inhibitor (uh-ROH-muh-tayz in-HIH-bih-ter): a drug that prevents the formation of estradiol, a female hormone, by interfering with an aromatase enzyme. Aromatase inhibitors are used as a type of hormone therapy for postmenopausal women who have hormone–dependent breast cancer.

axillary (AX-ill-air-ee) lymph node: a lymph node in the armpit.

axillary (AX-ill-air-ee) lymph node dissection (ALND): removal of the lymph nodes in the armpit (axillary nodes). They are examined under a microscope to determine whether they contain cancer. *See also* lymph nodes.

benign: not cancerous.

benign tumor: an abnormal growth that is not cancer and does not spread to other areas of the body.

biopsy (BUY-op-see): the removal of a sample of tissue to see whether cancer cells are present. There are several kinds of biopsies. *See also* surgical biopsy, needle biopsy, stereotactic needle biopsy, incisional biopsy.

bisphosphonates: drugs that are sometimes given to cancer patients whose disease has spread to the bones. When injected into a vein or taken by mouth, bisphosphonates can slow the breakdown of bone, lower the rate of bone fractures, and alleviate bone pain.

blood tumor marker: a substance that can be found in the blood when cancer is present. There are many different types of tumor markers.

blood vessel: a tube through which the blood circulates in the body. Blood vessels include a network of arteries, arterioles, capillaries, venules, and veins.

bone marrow: the soft tissue in the hollow center of some bones of the body that produces new blood cells. Bone marrow is often affected by chemotherapy. *See also* platelet, red blood cells, white blood cells.

bone scan: an imaging method that gives important information about the bones, including the location of cancer that may have spread to the bones. It can be done as an outpatient procedure and is painless, except for the needle stick when a low-dose radioactive substance is injected into a vein. Special pictures are taken to see where the radioactivity collects, pointing to an abnormality.

brachial plexopathy (BRAKE-ee-ul pleks-AH-puh-thee): a condition marked by numbness, tingling, pain, weakness, or limited movement in the arm or hand. It is caused by an impairment of the brachial plexus, a network of nerves that affect the arm and hand.

brachytherapy (brake-ee-THAYR-uh-pee): internal radiation treatment given by placing radioactive material directly into the tumor or close to it. Also called interstitial radiation therapy or seed implantation. *Compare with* external beam radiation therapy.

BRCA1: a gene that when damaged (mutated) places a woman at much greater risk of developing breast and/or ovarian cancer, compared with women who do not have the mutation.

BRCA2: a gene that when damaged (mutated) puts the carrier at a much higher risk for developing breast cancer and/or ovarian cancer than the general population.

breast: a glandular organ located on the chest. The breast is made up of connective tissue, fat, and breast tissue that contains the glands that can make milk. Also called mammary gland.

breast-conserving surgery: surgery to remove breast cancer and a small amount of normal tissue around the cancer (margin), without removing any other part of the breast. The lymph nodes under the arm may be removed. Radiation therapy is often administered after the surgery. This method is also called lumpectomy, segmental excision, limited breast surgery, or tylectomy. *See also* lymph nodes. *Compare with* mastectomy.

breast form: an artificial body part worn either inside the bra or attached to the body to simulate the appearance and feel of a natural breast. *Compare with* breast reconstruction.

breast implant: a sac used to increase breast size or restore the shape of the breast after mastectomy. The sac is filled with silicone gel (a synthetic material) or sterile saltwater (saline).

breast reconstruction: surgery done to rebuild the breast after mastectomy. A breast implant or the patient's own tissue is used. If desired, the nipple and areola may also be recreated. Reconstruction can be done at the time of mastectomy (immediate reconstruction) or any time later (delayed reconstruction). *Compare with* breast form.

breast self-examination (BSE): a method of checking one's own breasts for lumps or suspicious changes. BSE is an option for women in their 20s and older. The goals with BSE are to know what your breast tissue feels and looks like and to be able to report any breast changes to a doctor or nurse right away.

calcifications (kal-suh-fuh-KAY-shuns): tiny calcium deposits within the breast, either alone or in clusters, usually found by mammography. They are a sign of change within the breast that may need to be followed by more mammograms or by a biopsy. Calcifications may be caused by benign breast conditions or by breast cancer. The ones most closely linked to breast cancer are called **microcalcifications,** while the larger **macrocalcifications** are more often linked to benign changes.

cancer: cancer is not just one disease but a group of diseases. All forms of cancer cause cells in the body to change and grow out of control. Most types of cancer cells form a lump or mass called a tumor. The tumor can invade and destroy healthy tissue. Cells from the tumor can break away and travel to other parts of the body where they can continue to grow—a process called metastasis. When cancer spreads, it is still named after the part of the body where it started. For example, if breast cancer spreads to the lungs, it is still called breast cancer, not lung cancer.

Some cancers, such as blood cancers, do not form a tumor. A tumor is not always cancer; a tumor that is not cancer is called benign. Benign tumors do not grow and spread the way cancer does. Benign tumors are usually not a threat to life. Another word for cancerous is malignant.

cancer care team: the group of health care professionals who work together to diagnose, treat, and care for people with cancer. Whether the team is linked formally or informally, there is usually one person who coordinates care.

capsular contracture: scar tissue that forms around the implant and squeezes it. There are 4 grades of contracture (Grades I–IV) that range from normal and soft to hard, painful, and distorted.

carcinoma (kahr-si-NO-muh): any cancerous tumor that begins in the lining layer of organs. At least 80% of all cancers are carcinomas.

cell: the basic unit of which all living things are made. Cells replace themselves by splitting and forming new cells (mitosis). The processes that control the formation of new cells and the death of old cells are disrupted in cancer.

chemoprevention (key-mo-pre-VEN-shun): prevention or reversal of disease by using drugs, chemicals, vitamins, or minerals. Whereas this idea is not ready for widespread use, it is a very promising area of study.

chemotherapy (key-mo-THAYR-uh-pee): treatment with drugs to destroy cancer cells. Chemotherapy is often used, either alone or with surgery or radiation, to treat cancer that has spread or recurred, or when there is a strong chance that it could recur.

clinical breast examination (CBE): an examination of the breasts done by a health professional such as a doctor or nurse. Clinical breast exams are recommended every 3 years for women in their 20s and 30s, and every year for women age 40 and older.

clinical stage: an estimate of the extent of cancer based on physical exam, biopsy results, and imaging tests. *See also* pathologic stage, staging.

clinical trials: research studies to test new drugs or other treatments to compare current, standard treatments with others that may be better. Before a new treatment is used on people, it is studied in the laboratory. If laboratory studies suggest the treatment will work, the next step is to test its value for patients. These human studies are called clinical trials. The main questions the researchers want to answer are these:

- Does this treatment work?
- Does it work better than what we're currently using?
- What side effects does it cause?
- Do the benefits outweigh the risks?
- Which patients are most likely to find this treatment helpful?

comedocarcinoma: a form of breast cancer in which plugs of necrotic malignant cells may be expressed from the ducts. *See* necrosis.

complementary therapy (complementary medicine): treatment used in addition to standard therapy. Some complementary therapies may help relieve certain symptoms of cancer, relieve side effects of standard cancer therapy, or improve a patient's sense of well-being. The American Cancer Society recommends that patients considering the use of any alternative or complementary therapies discuss these therapies with their cancer care team, since many of these treatments are unproven and some can be harmful. *Compare with* alternative therapy.

computed tomography (to-MAHG-ruh-fee): an imaging test in which many x-rays are taken of a part of the body from different angles. These images are combined by a computer to produce cross-sectional pictures of internal organs. Except for the injection of a contrast dye (needed in some but not all cases), this is a painless procedure that can be done in an outpatient clinic. It is often referred to as "CT" or "CAT" scanning.

cone views with magnification: enlarging a section (or sections) of a mammogram film, so that the doctor can visualize the area more clearly.

control group: in research or clinical trials, the group that does not receive the treatment being tested. The group may get a placebo or sham treatment, or it may receive standard therapy. Also called the comparison group. *See also* clinical trials.

core needle biopsy: *see* needle biopsy.

Cowden syndrome: an inherited condition characterized by lesions that form on various organs, especially in the breast, thyroid, colon, skin, oral mucosa, and intestines. Cowden syndrome is associated with a higher risk for malignancies to develop in the organs involved. Also called Cowden disease.

CT scan or CAT scan: *see* computed tomography.

cyst (sist): a closed cavity in the body filled with fluid or semisolid material.

deep inferior epigastric artery perforator (DIEP) flap: a type of flap procedure that uses fat and skin from the same area as in the TRAM flap, but does not use the muscle to form the breast mound.

deoxyribonucleic (dee-ox-ee-rie-bo-noo-KLAY-ik) acid: *see* DNA.

detection: finding disease. Early detection means that the disease is found at an early stage, before it has grown large or spread to other sites.

diethylstilbestrol (DES): a man-made form of estrogen. Taking this drug during pregnancy may put women at a slightly higher risk of breast cancer.

digital mammogram: a method of storing an x-ray of the breast as a computer image rather than on the usual x-ray film. Digital mammography can be combined with computer-aided detection (CAD), a process in which the radiologist uses a computer program to help interpret the mammogram. Also known as full-field digital mammogram (FFDM). *See also* mammogram.

dimpling: a pucker or indentation of the skin. On the breast, it may be a sign of cancer.

diploid: *see* ploidy.

DNA: deoxyribonucleic acid. DNA is the genetic "blueprint" found in the nucleus of each cell. It holds genetic information on cell growth, division, and function.

duct: a hollow passage for gland secretions. In the breast, milk passes from the lobule (which makes the milk) through the ducts to the nipple.

ductal carcinoma (DUK-tal kahr-si-NO-muh): the most common type of breast cancer. It begins in the cells that line the milk ducts in the breast.

ductal carcinoma in situ (DUK-tal kahr-si-NO-muh in SIGH-too) (DCIS): cancer that starts in cells in the milk passages (ducts) and does not break through the duct walls into the nearby tissue. This is a highly curable form of breast cancer that is treated with surgery or surgery plus radiation therapy. Also called intraductal carcinoma.

ductal lavage (DUK-tal luh-VAZH): a method used to collect cells from milk ducts in the breast. A hair-size catheter (tube) is inserted into the nipple, and a small amount of salt water is released into the duct. The water picks up breast cells and is removed. The cells are checked under a microscope. Ductal lavage may be used in addition to clinical breast examination and mammography to detect breast cancer.

ductogram: a test in which a fine plastic tube is inserted into the nipple and contrast dye injected to outline the shape of the duct. X-rays are then taken to see if there is a mass. Also called a galactogram.

epithelial (ep-ih-THEE-lee-ul) cells: cells that line the internal and external surfaces of the body.

estrogen (ES-truh-jin): a female sex hormone produced mainly by the ovaries, and in smaller amounts by the adrenal glands. In women, levels of estrogen and other hormones work together to regulate the development of secondary sex characteristics, including breasts; regulate the monthly cycle of menstruation; and prepare the body for fertilization and reproduction. In breast cancer, estrogen may promote the growth of cancer cells. *See also* estrogen replacement therapy, hormone therapy.

estrogen receptors: *see* hormone receptor.

estrogen replacement therapy (ERT): the use of estrogen from sources other than the body. Estrogen may be administered after a woman's body no longer makes its own supply. This type of hormone therapy is often used to relieve symptoms of menopause in women who no longer have a uterus. It has also been shown to help protect against bone thinning (osteoporosis). Since estrogen nourishes some types of breast cancer, scientists are working on the question of whether ERT increases breast cancer risk. ERT probably will be shown to not increase the risk of breast cancer very much, if at all, especially if used for a relatively short period of time. But some studies have shown that it may increase the risk of stroke.

excisional biopsy: *see* surgical biopsy.

external beam radiation therapy (EBRT): radiation that is focused from a source outside the body on the area affected by the cancer. It is much like getting a diagnostic x-ray, but for a longer time and at a higher dose. Radiation to the breast can be delivered from outside the body in different ways. *Compare with* brachytherapy.

fatigue (fuh-TEEG): a common symptom during cancer treatment, a bone-weary exhaustion that doesn't get better with rest. For some, this condition can last for some time after treatment.

FDA: *see* U.S. Food and Drug Administration.

fibroadenoma (fi-bro-ad-un-O-muh): a breast tumor made of fibrous and glandular tissue that is not cancer. On a clinical breast exam or breast self-exam, it usually feels like a firm, round, smooth lump. Fibroadenomas usually occur in young women.

fibrocystic (fi-bro-SIS-tick) changes: certain changes in the breast that are not caused by cancer. Symptoms are breast swelling or pain. The breasts often feel lumpy or nodular. Because these signs sometimes resemble breast cancer, more tests may be needed to show that there is no cancer. Also called fibrocystic disease.

fine needle aspiration (FNA): *see* needle biopsy.

first-degree relative: a parent, sibling, or child. *Compare with* second-degree relative.

five (5)-year survival rate: the percentage of people with a specific cancer who are expected to survive 5 years or longer with the disease. Five-year survival rates have some drawbacks. Although the rates are based on the most recent information available, they may include data from patients treated several years earlier. Advances in cancer treatment often occur quickly. Five-year survival rates, while statistically valid, may not reflect these advances and should not be seen as a predictor in an individual case. *Compare with* relative five (5)-year survival rate.

free flap: surgery in which the tissue for reconstruction is moved entirely from another area of the body and the blood and nerve supplies are surgically reattached with special microscopes.

full-field digital mammogram (FFDM): *see* digital mammogram.

gadolinium (GA-duh-LIH-nee-um): a metal element that is used in magnetic resonance imaging (MRI) and other imaging methods. It is a contrast agent that helps reveal abnormal tissue in the body during an imaging procedure.

galactogram: *see* ductogram.

gene: a segment of DNA that contains information on hereditary characteristics such as hair color, eye color, and height, as well as susceptibility to certain diseases. *See also* DNA.

genetic counseling: the process of counseling people who may have a gene that makes them more susceptible to cancer. The purpose of the counseling is to help them decide whether they wish to be tested, to explore what the genetic test results might mean, and to support them before and after the test.

genetic risk factor: a risk factor that is inherited from a parent. A risk factor is anything that increases a person's chance of getting a disease such as cancer. Risk factors can be lifestyle-related or environmental, or genetic (inherited). Having a risk factor, or several risk factors, does not mean that a person will get the disease. Most cancers are not caused by genetic risk factors. If a patient has several family members with cancer, however, genetic testing may be considered. *See also* risk factor.

genetic testing: tests performed to determine whether a person has certain gene changes known to increase cancer risk. Such testing is not recommended for everyone, but specifically for individuals with specific types of family history. Genetic counseling should be part of the process.

glandular tissue: tissue that makes or secretes a substance.

gluteal free flap: a newer type of flap procedure that uses tissue and muscle from the buttocks to create the breast shape.

grade: the grade of a cancer reflects how abnormal it looks under the microscope. There are several grading systems for breast cancer, and each grading system divides cancer into those with the greatest abnormality, the least abnormality, and those in between. Grading is done by a pathologist who examines the tissue from the biopsy.

Grading is important because higher-grade cancers tend to grow and spread more quickly, and have a worse prognosis (outlook). Along with the cancer's stage, the grade is used to help determine the best treatment options. A cancer's **nuclear grade** is based on features of the central part of its cells, the nucleus. The **histologic grade** is based on features of individual cells as well as how the cells are arranged together. The histologic tumor grade can also be known as Bloom-Richardson grade, Scarff-Bloom-Richardson grade, or Elston-Ellis grade. *See also* stage, staging.

hand-foot syndrome: a condition marked by pain, swelling, numbness, tingling, or redness of the hands or feet. It sometimes occurs as a side effect of certain anticancer drugs.

helical CT: *see* spiral CT.

hematoma (he-muh-TOE-muh): a collection of blood outside a blood vessel caused by a leak or injury. A hematoma that occurs in the breast after injury or after surgery may feel like a lump.

HER2 gene: a gene that produces a type of receptor that helps cells grow. This receptor is present in very small amounts on the outer surface of normal breast cells. About 25% to 30% of breast cancers have too many of these receptors. These cancers tend to be more aggressive. They may respond to treatment with trastuzumab (Herceptin), a monoclonal antibody that attaches to the HER2 receptor. *See also* oncogenes.

histologic tumor grade: *see* grade.

Hodgkin disease (HOJ-kin dih-ZEEZ): a cancer of the immune system that is marked by the presence of a type of cell called the Reed-Sternberg cell. The two major types of Hodgkin disease are classic Hodgkin lymphoma and nodular lymphocyte–predominant Hodgkin lymphoma. Symptoms include the painless enlargement of lymph nodes, spleen, or other immune tissue. Other symptoms include fever, weight loss, fatigue, or night sweats. Also called Hodgkin lymphoma.

hormone: a chemical substance released into the body by the endocrine glands, such as the thyroid, adrenal glands, or ovaries. Hormones travel through the bloodstream and set in motion various body functions. For example, prolactin, which is produced in the pituitary gland, begins and continues milk production in the breast after childbirth. *See also* estrogen, progesterone.

hormone receptor: a protein on the surface of a cell to which a specific hormone binds. The hormone causes many changes to take place in the cell.

hormone replacement therapy (HRT): a therapy in which hormones are given to women after menopause to replace the hormones no longer produced by the body. Also called PHT (postmenopausal hormone therapy).

hormone therapy (HT): treatment with hormones, with drugs that interfere with hormone production or hormone action, or the surgical removal of hormone-producing glands to kill cancer cells or slow their growth. The most commonly used hormone therapy for breast cancer is the drug tamoxifen. Other hormone therapies include megestrol, aminoglutethimide, androgens, and surgical removal of the ovaries (oophorectomy).

hospice: a special kind of care for people in the final phase of illness, their families, and caregivers. The care may take place in the patient's home or in a home-like facility.

hot spots: areas of diseased bone that show up on bone scans. The hot spots can be bone metastasis, but they may also signify arthritis, infection, or other bone diseases.

hysterectomy (hiss-ter-EK-tuh-me): an operation to remove the uterus. Hysterectomy can be performed through a large incision in the abdomen (abdominal hysterectomy); through the vagina (vaginal hysterectomy); or by making a few very small incisions in the lower abdomen (laparoscopic hysterectomy). Removal of the ovaries (oophorectomy) may be done at the same time.

imaging tests: methods used to produce pictures of internal body structures. Some imaging methods used to help diagnose or stage cancer are x-rays, CT scans, magnetic resonance imaging (MRI), and ultrasound.

incisional biopsy: a surgical procedure in which tissue is removed and examined by a pathologist. The pathologist may study the tissue under a microscope or perform other tests. When an entire lump or suspicious area is removed, the procedure is called an excisional biopsy. When a sample of tissue or fluid is removed with a needle, the procedure is called a needle biopsy, core biopsy, or fine-needle biopsy (aspiration).

inflammatory breast cancer (IBC): a type of invasive breast cancer with spread to lymphatic vessels in the skin covering the breast. The skin of the affected breast is red, feels warm, and may thicken to look and feel like an orange peel. About 1% to 3% of invasive breast cancers are inflammatory carcinomas. Also called inflammatory carcinoma. *See also* invasive cancer, lymphatic system.

informed consent: a legal document that explains a course of treatment, the risks, benefits, and possible alternatives; the process by which patients agree to treatment.

infraclavicular (in-fruh-kluh-VICK-yuh-ler) lymph nodes: lymph nodes located beneath the clavicle (collar bone). *See also* lymph nodes, supraclavicular.

inherited (familial) cancer: cancer that originates from mutated genes that have been passed from parents to their offspring (children).

in situ (in SIGH-too): in place; localized and confined to one area. A very early stage of cancer.

internal mammary lymph nodes: *see* mammary lymph nodes.

intraductal carcinoma: *see* ductal carcinoma in situ.

intraductal papillomas: small, finger-like, noncancerous growths in the breast ducts that may cause a clear or bloody nipple discharge. These are most often found in women 45 to 50 years of age. A woman with a history of papillomas is at a slightly higher risk for breast cancer.

intraoperative radiation therapy: radiation treatment aimed directly at a tumor during surgery. Also called IORT.

intravenous (IV) line: a method of supplying fluids and medications by using a needle or a thin tube (called a catheter), which is inserted into a vein.

invasive breast cancer: cancer that spreads outside the breast tissue in which it began and invades other organs. *Compare with* noninvasive breast cancer.

invasive ductal carcinoma (IDC): cancer that starts in the milk passages (ducts) of the breast and then breaks through the duct wall and spreads into the fatty tissue of the breast. When it reaches this point, it can spread elsewhere in the breast, as well as to other parts of the body through the bloodstream and lymphatic system. Invasive ductal carcinoma is the most common type of breast cancer, accounting for about 80% of breast malignancies. Also known as infiltrating ductal carcinoma. *See also* lymphatic system.

invasive lobular carcinoma (ILC): a cancer that starts in the milk-producing glands (lobules) of the breast and then breaks through the lobule walls to spread into nearby fatty tissue. From this site, it may then spread elsewhere in the breast. About 10% of invasive breast cancers are invasive lobular carcinomas. It is often difficult to detect by physical examination or even by mammography. Also called infiltrating lobular carcinoma.

irradiation: the use of high-energy radiation from x-rays, gamma rays, neutrons, protons, and other sources to kill cancer cells and shrink tumors. Radiation may come from a machine outside the body (external beam radiation therapy), or it may come from radioactive material placed in the body near cancer cells (internal radiation therapy). Systemic irradiation uses a radioactive substance, such as a radiolabeled monoclonal antibody, that travels in the blood to tissues throughout the body. Also called radiation therapy and radiotherapy.

Ki-67 test: a test that measures the levels of a cancer antigen (Ki-67) in growing, dividing cells and serves as a good tumor marker. This test is done on a sample of tumor tissue, to help predict a patient's prognosis.

latissimus dorsi (LAT) flap: a procedure that tunnels muscle, fat, and skin from the upper back to the chest to create a breast mound.

leukemia (loo-KEE-mee-uh): cancer that starts in blood-forming tissue such as the bone marrow and causes large numbers of blood cells to be produced and enter the bloodstream.

Li-Fraumeni syndrome: a rare, inherited predisposition to multiple cancers, caused by an alteration in the p53 tumor suppressor gene.

lobular carcinoma (LAH-byuh-ler KAHR-si-NOH-muh): cancer that begins in the lobules (the glands that make milk) of the breast. Lobular carcinoma in situ (LCIS) is a condition in which abnormal cells are found only in the lobules. When cancer has spread from the lobules to surrounding tissues, it is invasive lobular carcinoma. LCIS does not become invasive lobular carcinoma very often, but having LCIS in one breast increases the risk of developing invasive cancer in either breast.

lobular carcinoma in situ (LAH-byuh-ler KAHR-si-NOH-muh in SIGH-too) (LCIS): although it is not a true cancer, LCIS is classified as a type of noninvasive cancer. It develops within the milk-producing glands (lobules) of the breast and does not break through the wall of the lobules. Researchers think that LCIS cells almost never progress to invasive lobular cancer. But having LCIS puts a woman at a higher risk of developing an invasive breast cancer later. For this reason, it's important for women with LCIS to have an annual mammogram and clinical breast exam. Also called lobular neoplasia. *See also* clinical breast examination, invasive lobular carcinoma, mammogram.

lobular neoplasia: *see* lobular carcinoma in situ.

lobules: milk-producing glands of the breast.

local therapy: treatment of cancer at its site, so that the rest of the body is not affected. Surgery and radiation therapy are examples of local therapy. *See also* systemic therapy.

lumpectomy (lum-PECK-tuh-me): surgery to remove the breast tumor and a small amount of the normal tissue around it. *See also* breast-conserving surgery.

lymph (limf): clear fluid that flows through the lymphatic vessels and contains cells known as lymphocytes. These cells are important in fighting infections and may also have a role in fighting cancer. *See also* lymphatic system, lymph nodes, lymphadenectomy.

lymphadenectomy (lim-fad-uh-NECK-tuh-me): surgical removal of one or more lymph nodes. After removal, the lymph nodes are examined by microscope to determine whether the cancer has spread. Also called lymph node dissection. *See also* lymphatic system, lymph, lymph nodes.

lymphatic system: a network of tissues and organs (including lymph nodes, spleen, thymus, and bone marrow) that produce and store lymphocytes (cells that fight infection) and the channels that carry the lymph fluid. The lymphatic system is an important part of the body's immune system, as its function is to fight infection. Invasive cancers sometimes penetrate the lymphatic vessels (channels) and spread (metastasize) to lymph nodes. *See also* lymph, lymph nodes, lymphadenectomy.

lymphatic vessel: a thin vessel (or tube) that carries lymph and white blood cells. *See also* lymph, lymphatic system.

lymphedema (limf-uh-DEE-muh): swelling due to a collection of excess fluid in the arms or legs. This may happen after the lymph nodes and vessels are removed or are injured by radiation, or it can happen many years after treatment. It may also happen when a tumor disrupts normal fluid drainage. Lymphedema can persist and interfere with activities of daily living. *See also* lymphatic system, lymph nodes.

lymph nodes: small, bean-shaped collections of immune system tissue such as lymphocytes, found along lymphatic vessels. They remove cell waste, germs, and other harmful substances from lymph. They help fight infections and also have a role in fighting cancer, although cancers sometimes spread through lymph nodes. Also called lymph glands. *See also* lymph, lymphatic system, lymphadenectomy.

macrocalcifications: *see* calcifications.

magnetic resonance imaging (MRI): a method of taking pictures of the inside of the body. Instead of using x-rays,

MRI uses a powerful magnet to send radio waves through the body. The images appear on a computer screen, as well as on film. Like x-rays, the procedure is physically painless, but some people may feel confined inside the MRI machine.

malignant: cancerous.

malignant tumor: a mass of cancer cells that may invade surrounding tissues or spread (metastasize) to distant sites in the body. *See also* tumor, metastasis.

mammary lymph nodes: lymph nodes that are near the sternum or breastbone, inside the chest. *See* lymph nodes.

mammogram, mammography: an x-ray of the breast; a way to find breast cancers that cannot be felt. Mammograms are done with a special type of x-ray machine that is used only for this purpose. A mammogram can show a developing breast tumor before it is large enough to be felt by a woman or even by a highly skilled health care professional. A **screening mammogram** is used to help find breast cancer early in women without any lumps or symptoms. A **diagnostic mammogram** helps the doctor learn more about breast masses that have been found by clinical breast exam, or the cause of other breast symptoms.

margin: the edge of the cancerous tissue or lump removed during surgery. A negative surgical margin is a sign that no cancer was left behind. A positive surgical margin means that cancer cells are found at the outer edge of the removed sample and is usually a sign that some cancer is still in the body.

mass: a lump or tumor, which may or may not be cancer.

mastectomy: surgery to remove all or part of the breast and sometimes other tissue. There are different types of mastectomy:
   Extended radical mastectomy removes the breast, skin, nipple, areola, chest muscles (pectoral major and minor), and all axillary and internal mammary lymph nodes on the same side.

Halsted radical mastectomy removes the breast, skin, nipple, areola, both pectoral muscles, and all axillary lymph nodes on the same side.

Modified radical mastectomy removes the breast, skin, nipple, areola, and most of the axillary lymph nodes on the same side, leaving the chest muscles intact.

Nipple-sparing mastectomy is surgery to remove internal breast tissue. The nipple and skin are left intact.

Partial mastectomy removes less than the whole breast, taking only the part of the breast in which the cancer occurs and a margin of healthy breast tissue surrounding the tumor.

Prophylactic mastectomy is a mastectomy done before any evidence of cancer can be found, to prevent cancer. This procedure is sometimes recommended for women at very high risk of breast cancer.

Quadrantectomy is a partial mastectomy in which the quarter of the breast that contains a tumor is removed.

Radical mastectomy removes the entire breast, axillary lymph nodes, and the chest wall muscles under the breast.

Segmental mastectomy is a partial mastectomy.

Simple mastectomy or **total mastectomy** removes only the breast and areola.

Skin-sparing mastectomy leaves as much of the breast skin as possible to improve the way the reconstructed breast looks.

mastitis: an infection in the breast that results in swelling, pain, warmth, and redness. Mastitis most commonly occurs in women who are breastfeeding.

menopausal hormone therapy (MHT): *see* hormone replacement therapy.

menopause (MEN-uh-paws): the time in a woman's life when monthly cycles of menstruation stop and hormone production by the ovaries decreases. Menopause usually occurs naturally when a woman is in her late 40s or early 50s (the average age is 51 years), but it can also be caused by surgical removal of both ovaries or by some chemotherapies that destroy ovarian function. Women who are past menopause are called menopausal or postmenopausal. Women who are still menstruating are called premenopausal. Those who have begun to have signs of menopause, but have not completely stopped menstruating are said to be perimenopausal.

metastasis (meh-TAS-tuh-sis): cancer cells that have spread to one or more sites elsewhere in the body, often by way of the lymphatic system or bloodstream. Regional metastasis is cancer that has spread to the lymph nodes, tissues, or organs close to the primary site. Distant metastasis is cancer that has spread to organs or tissues that are farther away (such as when breast cancer spreads to the bones or liver). *See also* primary site, lymph nodes, lymphatic system.

metastasize: the spread of cancer cells from one part of the body to another.

metastatic (met-uh-STAT-ick) cancer: a way to describe cancer that has spread from the primary site (where it started) to other structures or organs, nearby or far away (distant). *See also* primary site, metastasis.

microcalcifications: *see* calcifications.

modified radical mastectomy: *see* mastectomy.

monoclonal (ma-nuh-KLO-nuhl) antibody: a type of antibody manufactured in the laboratory. Monoclonal antibodies are designed to lock onto specific antigens (substances that can be recognized by the immune system). Monoclonal antibodies that have been attached to chemotherapy drugs or radioactive substances are being studied for their potential to seek out antigens unique to cancer cells and go directly to the cancer, thus killing the cancer cells and not harming healthy tissue. Monoclonal antibodies are also often used to help detect and classify cancer cells under a microscope. Other studies are being done to determine whether radioactive atoms attached to monoclonal antibodies can be used in imaging tests to detect and locate small groups of cancer cells. *See* antibody, antigen.

MRI: *see* magnetic resonance imaging.

mutation (myoo-TAY-shun): any change in the DNA of a cell. Mutations may be caused by mistakes during cell division, or they may be caused by exposure to DNA-damaging agents in the environment. Mutations can be harmful, beneficial, or have no effect. If they occur in cells that make eggs or sperm, they can be inherited; if mutations occur in other types of cells, they are not inherited. Certain mutations may lead to cancer or other diseases.

necrosis: the death of living tissues. Necrotic refers to tissue that has died.

needle biopsy: removal of fluid, cells, or tissue with a needle for examination under a microscope. There are 2 types: **fine needle aspiration (FNA)** and **core biopsy**. FNA uses a thin needle to draw up (aspirate) fluid or small tissue fragments from a cyst or tumor. A core needle biopsy uses a thicker needle to remove a cylindrical sample of tissue from a tumor.

neoadjuvant (nee-oh-AJ-oo-vunt) therapy: treatment given before the main treatment. *Compare with* adjuvant therapy.

neuropathy: nerve abnormality or damage, which causes numbness, tingling, pain, muscle weakness, or even swelling. It may be caused by injury, infection, disease (cancer, diabetes, kidney failure, or poor nutrition, for example), or by drugs. Peripheral neuropathy is a type of neuropathy that starts in nerves farthest away from the brain, such as the hands and feet.

nipple: the tip of the breast; the pigmented projection in the middle of the areola. The nipple contains the opening of milk ducts from the breast.

nipple aspiration: the collection of fluid containing cells from the lining of the milk ducts. The fluid is collected using gentle suction from a device similar to the breast pumps used by nursing women.

nipple discharge: any fluid coming from the nipple. It may be clear, milky, bloody, tan, gray, or green. In a nipple discharge examination, fluid is collected and examined under the microscope to determine whether any cancer cells are present.

nipple retraction: a turning inward of the nipple.

nipple-sparing mastectomy: *see* mastectomy.

non-Hodgkin lymphoma (NHL): a cancer of the lymphatic system.

noninvasive breast cancer: cancer that has not spread outside the breast tissue in which it began. *Compare with* invasive breast cancer, metastatic cancer.

nonproliferative lesions: conditions that are not associated with overgrowth of breast tissue and do not appear to affect breast cancer risk.

nonsteroidal anti-inflammatory drug: a drug that decreases fever, swelling, pain, and redness. Also called NSAID.

NSAID: *see* nonsteroidal anti-inflammatory drug.

nuclear grade: *see* grade.

oncogenes: genes that promote cell growth and multiplication. These genes are normally present in all cells. But oncogenes may undergo changes that activate them, causing cells to grow too quickly and form tumors.

oncoplastic surgery: the combination of surgery for cancer treatment and plastic surgery intended to remodel, repair, or restore body parts, especially by the transfer of tissue.

oophorectomy (oh-oh-foh-REK-toh-mee): surgery to remove one or both ovaries.

osteoclasts: large bone cells that break down and remove bone tissue.

osteonecrosis: the destruction and death of bone tissue.

osteoporosis: a condition that is marked by a decrease in bone mass and density, causing bones to become fragile.

ovarian ablation: a process that uses drugs or surgery to shut down the ovaries, which makes women postmenopausal and may allow some hormone therapies to work better.

p53: an important tumor suppressor gene that is not working properly in many cancers. The protein that this gene makes (also called p53) normally causes damaged cells to die. Mutations, or changes, in this gene can be inherited or they can occur during a person's life. When they do occur, they can increase risk of getting many types of cancer. *See* mutation, tumor suppressor gene.

Paget (PA-jet) disease of the nipple (formerly called Paget's disease): a rare form of breast cancer that begins in the milk ducts and spreads to the skin of the nipple and areola, which may cause oozing or look crusted, scaly, or red. The outlook is usually better if these nipple changes are the only sign of breast disease and no lump can be felt. *See* duct, nipple.

palliative (PAL-ee-uh-tiv) treatment: treatment that relieves symptoms, such as pain, but is not expected to cure the disease. Its main purpose is to improve the patient's quality of life. Sometimes chemotherapy and radiation are used as palliative treatments.

partial (segmental) mastectomy: *see* mastectomy

pathologic stage: an estimate of the extent of cancer by direct study of the samples removed during surgery. *See also* clinical stage, staging.

pectoral muscles: muscles attached to the front of the chest wall and upper arms. The larger one is called pectoralis major, and the smaller one is called pectoralis minor. Because these muscles are next to the breast, breast cancer may spread to them, although this rarely happens.

pedicle flap: tissue that is surgically removed, but the blood vessels remain attached and are tunneled from the original site to the area where the tissue is to be attached.

PET scan: *see* positron emission tomography.

platelet (PLATE-uh-let): a part of the blood that plugs up holes in blood vessels after an injury. Chemotherapy can cause a drop in the platelet count, a condition called thrombocytopenia that carries a risk of excessive bleeding.

ploidy (ploy-dee): a measure of the amount of DNA within a cell. Ploidy is a marker that helps predict how quickly a cancer is likely to spread. Cancers with the same amount of DNA as normal cells are called **diploid**, and those with either more or less than that amount are **aneuploid**. Patients with diploid cancers have longer disease-free intervals and a better prognosis, but about 2 of 3 breast cancers are aneuploid. This test is done by using lasers and computers, a process called flow cytometry.

positron emission tomography (PAHS-ih-trahn ee-MISH-uhn toh-MAHG-ruh-fee) (PET): a PET scan creates an image of the body (or of biochemical events) after the injection of a very low dose of a radioactive form of a substance such as glucose (sugar). The scan computes the rate at which the tumor is using the sugar. In general, high-grade tumors use more sugar than normal and low-grade tumors. PET scans are especially useful in taking images of the brain, although they are becoming more widely used to find the spread of cancer of the breast, colon, rectum, ovary, or lung. PET scans may also be used to see how well the tumor is responding to treatment.

postmenopausal hormone therapy (PHT): *see* hormone replacement therapy.

primary site: the place where cancer begins. Primary cancer is usually named after the organ in which it starts. For example, cancer that starts in the breast is always breast cancer even if it spreads (metastasizes) to other organs, such as the lungs, bones, and liver.

progesterone (pro-JES-ter-own): a female sex hormone released by the ovaries during every menstrual cycle to prepare the uterus for pregnancy and the breasts for milk production. *See also* hormone, estrogen.

progesterone receptors: *see* hormone receptor.

prognosis (prog-NO-sis): a prediction of the course of disease; the outlook for the chances of survival.

proliferative (pro-lih-fer-uh-tiv) lesions with atypia:
excessive growth of cells in the ducts or lobules of the
breast tissue where the cells deviate from normal cells
when examined under the microscope. *See* duct, lobules.
Compare with proliferative lesions without atypia.

proliferative (pro-lih-fer-uh-tiv) lesions without atypia:
excessive growth of cells in the ducts or lobules of the
breast tissue where the cells do not deviate from normal
cells when examined under the microscope. *See* duct,
lobules. *Compare with* proliferative lesions with atypia.

prosthesis (pros-THEE-sis): an artificial part used to
replace or improve the function of a body part. A breast
form is an example of a prosthesis.

quadrantectomy: *see* mastectomy.

quality of life: overall enjoyment of life, which includes a
person's sense of well-being and ability to do the things that
are important to him or her.

radiation (RAY-dee-AY-shun): energy released in the form
of particles or electromagnetic waves. Common sources of
radiation include radon gas, cosmic rays from outer space,
medical x-rays, and energy given off by a radioisotope.

radiation therapy: treatment with high-energy rays (such
as x-rays) to kill or shrink cancer cells. The radiation may
come from outside of the body (external radiation) or
from radioactive materials placed directly in the tumor
(brachytherapy or internal radiation). Radiation therapy
may be used as the main treatment for a cancer, to reduce
the size of a cancer before surgery, or to destroy any
remaining cancer cells after surgery. In advanced cancer
cases, it may also be used as palliative treatment. *See also*
external beam radiation therapy, brachytherapy, palliative
treatment.

radical mastectomy: *see* mastectomy.

randomized or randomization: a process used in clinical
trials that uses chance to assign participants to different
groups that compare treatments. Randomization means

that each person has an equal chance of being in either the treatment or comparison groups. This helps reduce the chance of bias in the results that might happen, if, for example, the healthiest people all were assigned to a particular treatment group. *See also* control group, clinical trials.

reconstruction: *see* breast reconstruction.

recurrence: the return of cancer after treatment. **Local recurrence** means that the cancer has come back at the same place as the original cancer. **Regional recurrence** means that the cancer has come back after treatment in the lymph nodes near the primary site. **Distant recurrence**, also known as metastatic recurrence, is when cancer metastasizes after treatment to distant organs or tissues (such as the lungs, liver, bone marrow, or brain). *See also* primary site, metastasis, metastasize.

red blood cells: blood cells that contain hemoglobin, the substance that carries oxygen to all of the cells of the body.

reexcision: a second surgery to remove remaining cancer. This may be done if cancer cells are found at the edge of surgically removed tissue. *See* margin.

relative five (5)-year survival rate: the percentage of people with a specific cancer who have not died of it within 5 years. This number is different from the 5-year survival rate in that it does not include people who have died of unrelated causes.

risk factor: anything that affects a person's chance of getting a disease such as cancer. Different cancers have different risk factors. For example, unprotected exposure to strong sunlight is a risk factor for skin cancer; smoking is a risk factor for lung, mouth, larynx, and other cancers. Some risk factors, such as smoking, can be controlled. Others, like a person's age, cannot be changed.

S-phase fraction: a laboratory test that shows the percentage of cells that are replicating or reproducing their DNA. DNA replication is usually a sign that a cell is getting ready to split into 2 new cells. A low S-phase fraction is a sign that a tumor is slow-growing; a high S-phase fraction shows that the cells are dividing rapidly and the tumor is growing quickly. *See* DNA.

sarcoma (sar-KO-muh): a cancer starting in connective tissues, such as cartilage, fat, muscle, or bone. Several types of sarcoma (such as angiosarcoma, liposarcoma, and malignant phyllodes tumor) can develop in the breast, although this is rare.

scan: a study using either x-rays or radioactive isotopes to produce images of internal body organs.

scintimammography (SIN-tih-ma-MAH-gruh-fee): a breast imaging test that is used to detect cancer cells in the breasts of some women who have had abnormal mammograms, or who have dense breast tissue. It is not used for screening or as a substitute for a mammogram. With scintimammography, a woman receives an injection of a small amount of a radioactive substance called technetium 99, which is taken up by cancer cells, and a gamma camera is used to take pictures of the breasts.

screening: the search for disease, such as cancer, in people without symptoms. For example, screening measures recommended by the American Cancer Society for breast cancer include clinical breast exams and mammograms. Screening may also refer to coordinated programs in large populations.

second-degree relative: an aunt, uncle, grandparent, grandchild, niece, nephew, or half-sibling. *Compare with* first-degree relative.

sentinel lymph node biopsy (BUY-op-see): a diagnostic procedure involving the removal of the first lymph node to which cancer cells are likely to spread from the primary tumor. In some cases, there can be more than one sentinel lymph node. For this procedure, a radioactive substance or contrast dye is injected near the tumor. A scanner is then used to map the circulation of the substance through the primary (sentinel) node. The node is then removed and examined for the presence of cancer cells. *See also* lymph node.

seroma: a tumorlike collection in the tissues of the clear liquid part of the blood that remains after blood cells and clotting proteins have been removed.

skin-sparing mastectomy: *see* mastectomy.

spiral CT: a special scanner that takes cross-sectional pictures around the body. Also called helical CT. *See also* computed tomography,.

stage: the extent of a cancer in the body. *See* staging.

staging: the process of finding out whether cancer has spread and, if so, how far.
The TNM system, which is the most common system used to describe the stages of breast cancer, gives 3 key pieces of information:
- T refers to the size of the tumor
- N describes how far the cancer has spread to nearby lymph nodes
- M shows whether the cancer has spread (metastasized) to other organs of the body

Letters or numbers after the T, N, and M give more details about each of these factors. To make this information more clear, the TNM descriptions can be grouped together into a simpler set of stages, labeled with Roman numerals (usually from I to IV). In general, the lower the number, the less the cancer has spread. A higher number means a more serious cancer. The 2 types of staging are clinical staging and pathologic staging. *See also* clinical stage, pathologic stage.

stem cell transplant: a method of replacing immature blood-forming cells that were destroyed by cancer treatment. The stem cells are given to the person after treatment to help the bone marrow recover and continue producing healthy blood cells.

stereotactic needle biopsy: a method of needle biopsy that is useful in some cases where there are calcifications or a mass that can be seen on mammogram but cannot be felt. A computer maps the location of the mass to guide the placement of the needle. When this type of biopsy is done with a larger needle, it may be called a **stereotactic core needle biopsy**. *See also* needle biopsy.

stereotactic wire localization: a procedure used to guide a surgical breast biopsy when the lump is hard to find or when there is an area that looks suspicious on a mammogram. A thin hollow needle is placed into the breast, and computer images are taken to guide the needle to the area in question. A fine thin wire is inserted through the center of the needle. A small hook at the end of the wire keeps it in place. The hollow needle is then removed, and the surgeon uses the path of the wire as a guide to find the abnormal area to be removed. *See also* biopsy, mammogram, x-ray.

stroma: fatty and connective tissue.

supraclavicular (sue-pruh-cluh-VIK-you-lar) lymph nodes: lymph nodes just above the collarbone (clavicle). *See* lymph nodes.

surgical biopsy: a method of biopsy in which all or part of a lump is removed by a surgeon for examination. *See also* biopsy, stereotactic wire localization.

surgical margin: *see* margin.

systemic therapy: treatment that reaches and affects cells throughout the entire body; for example, chemotherapy.

tamoxifen: a drug used to prevent breast cancer in high-risk women; decrease the risk of getting invasive breast cancer in women with ductal cancer in situ (DCIS); help keep cancer from coming back after surgery, radiation, and chemotherapy; and treat advanced breast cancer. It is also used to treat other types of cancer and may be used for other conditions.

targeted therapy: treatment that attacks the part of cancer cells that makes them different from normal cells, as opposed to treatment that harms all cells. Targeted therapy tends to have fewer side effects than some standard treatments such as chemotherapy.

tissue: a collection of cells, united to perform a particular function in the body.

tissue expander: a balloon implanted under the skin and used to keep living tissues under tension. This causes new cells to form and stretches the tissue. The surgeon puts the expander beneath the skin where the breast should be and, over a period of weeks or months, injects a saline solution to slowly expand the overlaying skin to make space for an implant.

tissue flap reconstruction: tissue for reconstruction that is surgically removed from another area of the body. It can be a pedicle (left attached to its base and then tunneled under the skin) or free flap (cut free from its base and transplanted to the chest).

tomosynthesis: an imaging technique that produces a digital picture representing a detailed cross-section of tissue structures at a predetermined depth where the x-ray tube takes multiple low-dose exposures as it moves through a limited arc of motion.

total mastectomy: *see* mastectomy.

transducer: a device that converts one form of energy, such as pressure, temperature, or pulse, into another form of energy, often an electrical signal.

transverse rectus abdominis muscle (TRAM) flap: a procedure that uses tissue and muscle from the lower abdominal wall to reconstruct a breast mound. It can be a pedicle (left attached to its base and then tunneled under the skin) or free flap (cut free from its base and transplanted to the chest).

triple-negative breast cancer: a type of breast cancer, usually an invasive ductal carcinoma, in which the cells lack estrogen and progesterone receptors and do not have an excess of HER2 protein on their surfaces. Hormone therapy and drugs that target HER2 are not effective for treating this type of cancer. *See also* hormone receptor, hormone therapy, and HER2 gene.

tumor: an abnormal lump or mass of tissue. Tumors can be benign (noncancerous) or malignant (cancerous).

tumor necrosis: *see* necrosis.

tumor suppressor genes: genes that slow down cell division or cause cells to die at the appropriate time. Alterations of these genes can lead to too much cell growth and development of cancer.

ultrasound: an imaging method in which high-frequency sound waves are used to outline a part of the body. The sound wave echoes are picked up and displayed on a screen. Also called ultrasonography.

U.S. Food and Drug Administration (FDA): an agency of the United States Department of Health and Human Services. The FDA is responsible for regulating drugs, tobacco products, biological medical products, blood products, medical devices, and radiation-emitting devices, along with other products.

vascular endothelial growth factor (VAS-kyoo-ler EN-doh-THEE-lee-ul growth FAK-ter) (VEGF): a substance made by cells that stimulates new blood vessel formation.

white blood cells: cells that help defend the body against infections, which work as part of the immune system. This is one of many types of blood cells made in the bone marrow. Certain cancer treatments (especially chemotherapy) can reduce the number of these cells (a condition called neutropenia) and make a person more likely to get infections. *See also* bone marrow.

Women's Health Initiative (WHI): a very large prevention study in the United States established in 1991 to address the most common causes of death, disability, and impaired quality of life in postmenopausal women.

x-ray: one form of radiation that can be used at low levels to produce an image of the body on film or at high levels to destroy cancer cells.

Index

Books Published
by the American Cancer Society

Available everywhere books are sold and online at
http://www.cancer.org/bookstore

Information

The American Cancer Society: A History of Saving Lives

American Cancer Society's Complete Guide to Colorectal Cancer

American Cancer Society Complete Guide to Complementary & Alternative Cancer Therapies, Second Edition

American Cancer Society Complete Guide to Nutrition for Cancer Survivors: Eating Well, Staying Well During and After Cancer, Second Edition

Breast Cancer Clear & Simple: All Your Questions Answered

The Cancer Atlas (available in English, Spanish, French, and Chinese)

Cancer: What Causes It, What Doesn't

QuickFACTS™—Advanced Cancer

QuickFACTS™—Bone Metastasis

QuickFACTS™—Colorectal Cancer, Second Edition

QuickFACTS™—Lung Cancer

QuickFACTS™—Prostate Cancer, Second Edition

QuickFACTS™—Thyroid Cancer

The Tobacco Atlas, Third Edition (available in English, Spanish, French, and Chinese)

Day-to-Day Help

American Cancer Society's Guide to Pain Control: Understanding and Managing Cancer Pain, Revised Edition

Cancer Caregiving A to Z: An At-Home Guide for Patients and Families

Caregiving: A Step-By-Step Resource for Caring for the Person with Cancer at Home, Revised Edition

Get Better! Communication Cards for Kids & Adults

Kicking Butts: Quit Smoking and Take Charge of Your Health, Second Edition

Lymphedema: Understanding and Managing Lymphedema After Cancer Treatment

Social Work in Oncology: Supporting Survivors, Families and Caregivers

What to Eat During Cancer Treatment

When the Focus Is on Care: Palliative Care and Cancer

Emotional Support

Angels & Monsters: A child's eye view of cancer

Cancer in the Family: Helping Children Cope with a Parent's Illness

Chemo and Me: My Hair Loss Experience

Couples Confronting Cancer: Keeping Your Relationship Strong

Crossing Divides: A Couple's Story of Cancer, Hope, and Hiking Montana's Continental Divide

I Can Survive

The Survivorship Net: A Parable for the Family, Friends, and Caregivers of People with Cancer

What Helped Get Me Through: Cancer Survivors Share Wisdom and Hope

Just for Kids

Because . . . Someone I Love Has Cancer: Kids' Activity Book

Healthy Me: A Read-Along Coloring & Activity Book

Jacob Has Cancer: His Friends Want to Help

Kids' First Cookbook: Delicious-Nutritious Treats To Make Yourself!

Let My Colors Out

The Long and the Short of It: A Tale About Hair

Mom and the Polka-Dot Boo-Boo

Nana, What's Cancer?

No Thanks, but I'd Love to Dance

Our Dad Is Getting Better

Our Mom Has Cancer (hardcover)

Our Mom Has Cancer (paperback)

Our Mom Is Getting Better

What's Up with Bridget's Mom? Medikidz Explain Breast Cancer

What's Up with Richard? Medikidz Explain Leukemia

Prevention

The American Cancer Society's Healthy Eating Cookbook: A celebration of food, friendship, and healthy living, Third Edition

Celebrate! Healthy Entertaining for Any Occasion

Good for You! Reducing Your Risk of Developing Cancer

The Great American Eat-Right Cookbook: 140 Great-Tasting, Good-for-You Recipes

Healthy Air: A Read-Along Coloring & Activity Book (25 per pack: Tobacco avoidance)

Healthy Bodies: A Read-Along Coloring & Activity Book (25 per pack: Physical activity)

Healthy Food: A Read-Along Coloring & Activity Book (25 per pack: Nutrition)

National Health Education Standards: Achieving Excellence, Second Edition (available in paperback and on CD-ROM)

Reduce Your Cancer Risk